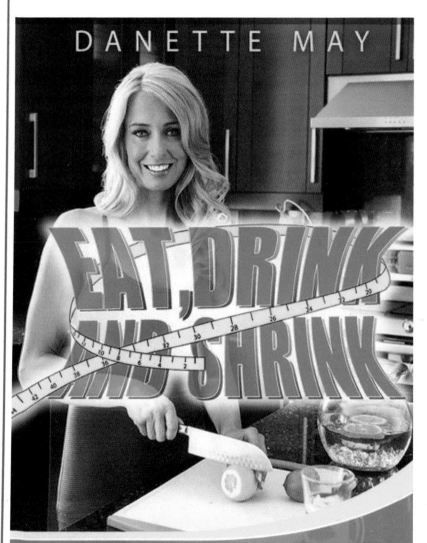

DANETTE MAY

EAT, DRINK AND SHRINK

Over 120 delicious, fat-burning recipes with only FIVE ingredients or less

ISBN 13: 978-0615937571
ISBN: 0615937578

Disclaimer and Terms of Use

The Author and Publisher have strived to be as accurate and complete as possible in the creation of this book. While all attempts have been made to verify information provided in this publication, the Author and Publisher assumes no responsibility for errors, omissions, or contrary interpretation of the subject matter herein. Any perceived slights of specific persons, peoples, or organizations are unintentional. In practical advice books, like anything else in life, there are no guarantees of results. Readers cautioned to rely on their own judgment about their individual circumstances to act accordingly.

This book is an educational guide that provides general health information. The materials in **Eat, Drink and Shrink** are "as is" and without warranties of any kind either express or implied.

The book's content is not a substitute for direct, personal, professional medical care and diagnosis. None of the diet plans or exercises (including products and services) mentioned in the book should be performed or otherwise used without clearance from your physician or health care provider. The information contained within is not intended to provide specific physical or mental health advice, or any other advice whatsoever, for any individual or company and should not be relied upon in that regard. We are not medical professionals and nothing in this book should be misconstrued to mean otherwise.

There may be risks associated with participating in activities mentioned in Eat, Drink and Shrink for people in poor health or with pre-existing physical or mental health conditions. Because these risks exist, you will not participate in such diet or exercise plans if you are in poor health or have a pre-existing mental or physical condition. If you choose to participate in these risks, you do so of your own free will and accord, knowingly and voluntarily assuming all risks associated with such dietary activities.

Eat, Drink and Shrink Acknowledgments

There are so many people to thank in my journey of bringing **Eat, Drink and Shrink** to life. I want to first thank my two precious girls who have tried every single one of the recipes, and would support me when I needed to spend time working. They have been patient and such an inspiration to me to ensure that I provide healthy tasty meals for families everywhere.

I want to thank Lululemon clothing for their donations and support, and Body Rock Sports Clothing for providing cute and comfortable sportswear for the cover of the Success Tracker. And I want to thank Darien Child for providing her home to shoot the cover of the book and for her continual friendship and support. I love you!

I want to thank all my clients who have worked with me! You have reached your goals and have been an inspiration to me. Seeing and hearing from every single one of you on your successes is what would keep driving me to push hard to get this program to the world. I love every single one of you and am thankful for your light in my life.

Finally I am thankful to a loving God who has been my pillar during the ups and downs in the creation of this product. I have felt God carrying me and supporting me in bringing this abundant program to you.

CONTENTS

Introduction

If you are reading this, then you want the body you see in your mind's eye, not the one you see in the mirror, or the one you have allowed to get beyond your control. I am here to let you know you can take back control. Sure, you've heard that statement before, but you have not heard it from me.

I know firsthand that this book can and will change your body, change your body's chemistry, change your attitude, and put you mentally, physically and emotionally in a state you probably haven't been in for a long time, if ever. This book is for you!

I wrote this book to eliminate excuses and help you create lasting weight loss results!

Repeatedly I have watched as we buy into these fad diets, or else we're handing over our hard-earned money for the latest, greatest diet pills on the market. I have watched many slight-of-hand performers create anxiety, deprivation, eventually weight loss, but at what sacrifice.

Only to have a Yo-Yo effect of gaining the weight right back. I see many people buying foods advertised on TV as low-fat, low-sugar and food supposed to help you lose weight, when in actuality these foods create more toxins in your body and leave you feeling more bloated and defeated than ever. I have watched as people limit their caloric intake to feel sluggish, "*hangry*" (hungry + angry) and on edge.

I have the tools to help!

I say, enough! I have the tools to help everyone feel energized and not deprived in the process of losing weight. I know how to get myself and thousands of others to lose weight, increase their energy, and eat frequently, all without feeling deprived. I know how to eliminate the excuse of *lack of time* when it comes to food prep, and I know how to keep the food budget to a minimum.

Hey, I'm a single mom; I'm sure like many of you. Being a single, working mother, I understand the value of time, money & energy! I wanted to create recipes that took 10-15 minutes or less to prepare, using the minimum of ingredients, while saving time and money at the grocery store. However, most importantly, I wanted to give my body, my children's bodies, and all of you the best nutrition guide to live an abundantly, energy rich life.

I personally do not like to cook or spend time in the kitchen. That said, I created over 120 recipes you can prepare, each with 5 ingredients or less, and they take 15 minutes or less to prepare! Nevertheless, the exciting part for me was creating fast, clean foods with delicious taste! My friends, family, and my children all enjoy eating these foods.

I do not like to prepare food, but I do enjoy eating it! The key to energized and lasting weight loss is to take the weight off and maintain it, all without feeling deprived. I say, "energized **weight loss**", because too many programs leave you feeling sluggish and on edge.

Scientific meal plans deliver results!

These recipes and the accompanying scientific meal plans deliver results. The scientific meal plan of eating throughout the day, with the right proportions, and the right fat burning food combinations, is the missing link in transforming your body for life!

The added highlight for me and one that gets me the most excited is knowing that I am helping thousands just like you, lose weight, gain energy, and transform in both body and mind with my scientific breakthrough meal plan and easy, delicious recipes. The recipes will give you what you need to transform and become the new you that you've always desired.

About me- Why I wrote this book!

I, like you, want to feel like I am contributing to "life" in some way! I felt like, if I was called to write this book and to give it to all of you, that it would flow easily and that I would be inspired to say the things that you need to hear to gain the tools, not only physically, but mentally as well.

I must say, my writings have spilled from me and I feel so "called" to share with you about the power of your mind in sabotaging your success! Most of you have tried lots. I mean lots, of different avenues to achieve the body of your dreams. You have tried and then for some reason end up in the same spot as you were in the beginning of your journey, some of you worse off than you were when you began.

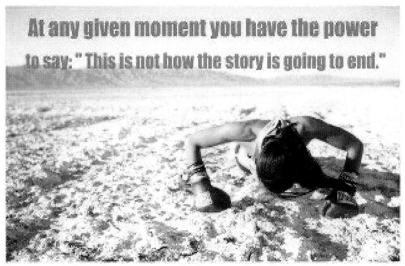

At any given moment you have the power to say: "This is not how the story is going to end."

I saw this picture, and instantly fell in love with the message. Despite what you may think, I completely understand how it feels to go through hard things, to awaken and wonder how my life took this extreme detour.

I, perhaps like you, wondered if I had the drive and determination to change my life story. In my case, the determination needed to write the remaining chapters of this book with zest, energy, passion, and purpose.

I want to share with you my personal struggles, not for you to feel sorry for me, but for you to understand that we all have been dealt our hand of cards. It is up to us to determine how we play them. Are we going to enjoy the game and play the best hand given to us?

We all have our own struggles and garbage. No one's garbage is bigger or smells worse than the next person's garbage – it is just garbage and it belongs to each of us. But one thing that rings loudest and most true in my mind (hence why I spend all my time writing and sharing with all of you), is all our garbage is more manageable when we keep our bodies as clean as possible through nutrition, exercise and positive self-talk!

I have heard every excuse imaginable as to why you are "different" than everyone else and you seem unable to reach your goals. Usually our goals are to look skinny and feel good in our clothes, when our "real" desires are centered on feeling confident with ourselves in every situation, naked, in clothes, when we speak, when we are with friends, with our family and with strangers.

We also want to feel like we have the energy to serve and to resonate our purpose in this world. **We all want to feel happy and to make positive progress in our lives.** We all know intuitively that it is a lot more difficult to feel inspired, to feel energetic, and to feel on point, when our bodies do not match up with our souls. Have you had one or more of these excuses in your life?

- I do not have enough time
- I work a full time job and have kids
- Eating healthy doesn't taste good
- My body has so many health problems that it has a harder time dropping the pounds
- My hormones are off, which creates weight gain
- I don't have a supportive husband, mom, dad, or children
- My body is just fat and I have tried everything and nothing works. Every time I start a program, crisis comes in our family and so I have to focus on other things

I understand these excuses because I have heard them and I have experienced many of them in my own life. As a trainer, I have studied various forms of fitness, muscle movements, and nutrition.

I have worked with thousands and have helped them see tremendous results, as I dived into their minds and helped conquer their eating and exercise patterns and their self-talk. It was not until I was dealt my hand of cards these past 6 years that I truly felt the effects of self-sabotage and the power of the mind to create excuses. Five years ago, I lost my son at birth. I experienced deep depression as my dreams of being a mother to a boy were vanished in an hours' worth of time.

The ride home is one of my most vivid memories. We went so slowly. I mean, you always drive home slow when you're first bringing home a baby, but we went really slowly without having the joy of bringing him with us. We drove slowly because we really didn't want to go home; there was no happiness, nothing to look forward to. We just had a baby but there was no baby in the car with us, but my whole body was telling me I had just had a baby.

My body literally craved him as I went through all the physical changes. It wanted to feed him, hold him, and it called out in pain for months, as I had to wait as these changes subsided. My body really hurt. Of course my milk came in and all of those internal feelings as a mom like the need to feed your baby- only I didn't have a child to feed, it was just a constant reminder that I no longer had my son.

I didn't know how to talk about it and I didn't know how to really deal with it. I was always the type that works out, **happy** and wanted to learn about nutrition, but I felt myself not wanting to do any of those things. I just wanted to stay in bed. It was my first encounter with true depression.

Not really knowing what to expect with depression. I had never dealt **with** it before. It took about a good three to four months for my body to really subside all those cravings of wanting this baby in my life and to deal with the physical and emotional changes. I still had that baby belly, and all those reminders, but no baby.

I didn't want to walk, I didn't want to exercise and I didn't! I just remember lying in bed and going, "I just need to walk around the block. Today, I will walk around the block." It was really hard. I remember thinking, "What is happening to me? Why can't I even walk around my block? Why don't I even want to walk around my block?"

I didn't feel like myself and I didn't even know who I was or what had happen to me, but I got on my shoes and I remember that walk. I remember the exact homes I passed and I remember this bird singing. It kind of sounds cliché, but I started to feel my chest like the emotions were coming up, but it was good. It was coming out.

I started to cry and I was walking and I remember thinking, "This is what is going to heal me. I need to share with the world that they need to move." Because just going through that and knowing that it was actually helping me heal, just this walk around the block was my step in my healing process, because it let my heart open.

I cried and released everything. I wasn't just holding it in anymore. The birds were singing to me. It was one of those moments for me. I knew I needed to heal and share healing, zest, being alive and healthy with the world! Every day I would start with the walk around the block because that's all I could do. I saw with each step of movement, how my heart was mending. It was an opening of understanding how movement/exercise releases depression & mends the soul.

Not long after that I was going through divorce, financial struggle, and the realization of being a "single" mom to two beautiful girls whom I love. All the excuses I heard my clients ring out, where raging in my head; depression, lack of time, exhaustion, and a whole array of emotions and fears flung at me. It was during this time, I "really" understood how this program could help many of you, too.

During this time, I emotionally wanted to curl up in bed, eat comfort foods, and not crawl out until the storm was over. Ok, I tried a couple days of it and it only spun me farther down. My face completely broke out due to stress, my neck was in chronic pain, and I could have easily gained weight during this time. I began in those days to lose hope. I wondered if I would live out my dreams. My body felt terrible, my mind was lethargic, and I was no use to anyone, especially my precious children. It was during this episode in my life that I began seeing with even clearer eyes the importance of eating clean and exercising daily.

Again it may sound cliché, but it was as if a voice was saying, "If I eat clean, that's going to actually help me have the energy to get through today." I chose to take the higher road and to write my own story. I decided each day was a new one. I decided I get to write on these pages, as I desire. I have choices, either to quit or take action.
Let me tell you, taking action is a whole lot easier when you have clean food in your system, adequate sleep, and stress reducing movement under your belt. When I have

worked out, gone for a walk/run, or gone to the gym, I always emerge feeling more hopeful about my future. I feel more ready to conquer. I am so grateful for these lessons. I am so grateful for healing, loving foods!

Napoleon Hill would say, "From out of chaos comes equal or greater good." I really felt like that. I felt like through my movement and eating clean, I was seeing that there was a purpose in it all!

We all know that we need to eat well. We all pretty much know the basics of good nutrition. We all know that we need to move and we all get a little bit motivated to do it when everything in our world is going perfectly or so called perfectly. I don't want to swear, but when the shit hits the fan, it's like that's the true test. That's actually when you need it the most, but it's the hardest time to actually implement those principles.

You are in charge of your life. You are the only one who gets to decide how it ends. Start writing on your pages today with hope, clarity and a renewed resolve to feed your body with the best and to move it for healing.

If you really want to fulfill your purpose and you really want to live a happy abundant life, then you need to remember that everyone is going to be dealt their cards, as I say. Everyone is going to have their hard times, everyone is, whatever that is: losing job, getting a divorce, someone dying that means a lot to you- everyone is going to have that moment. What gets you through that moment is really taking care of YOU and that's through proper nutrition and moving your body. That's how you're going to heal quicker and ultimately heal altogether.

It's not so much about how you look, I didn't write the book so everyone could look like a bikini model or to feel like a bikini model. (but if you eat from this plan, you will. :))Eating clean and moving is one piece in the whole puzzle of becoming your ultimate self. When you line that up, then every day you don't have to say, "I wish I could lose 20-30 pounds. If I lose 20-30 pounds, I would be happy." If-if-if, and using that as your anchor to not propel yourself to be your best self!

I know when someone feels good about himself or herself, each has more capacity to get out and enjoy nature, to enjoy his or her families and friends, and love more deeply. I know that feeling good about one's self creates healthier relationships with your spouse or partner, your family, friends, and associates. As your openness grows, oneness with others increases, and your satisfaction in all your relationships increases ten-fold.

In closing, you are in charge of your life. You are the only one who gets to decide how it ends.

Danette

Chapter One

Science behind Five Ingredients

Having been a fitness professional for over 13 years, an international speaker, leading health and fitness retreats, etc. I have worked with literally thousands of people. During this time, I have loved helping people get their "life" back on track by adopting a daily exercise & nutrition program.

I was helping many people, but I knew that I needed to reach out to even more! My dream was to create a program that anyone could do, at any age, any lifestyle, and in any place. I wanted to eliminate all the main excuses when it came to "life" and help millions of people from all lifestyles have a program they can maintain anywhere, at any stage, at any time to live active, healthy lives.

I wanted them to be able to enhance their relationships with not only their loved ones, but with others and within their own lives. That dream became a reality in Eat, Drink, & Shrink, which you hold in your hands today. And in the process, an amazing community called Forever Fit Challenge was also created to provide ongoing support, community, and health & fitness training.

This breakthrough scientific model of the **Eat, Drink and Shrink** recipe book and accompanying meal plans is exactly what you need to get your life back on track & start creating an abundance of health and fitness in your life, all while attaining the body of your dreams!

The **Eat, Drink and Shrink** recipes are based on the science of eating meals with five ingredients or less using fat-burning, clean & whole foods that taste delici9ous!

The science behind using five ingredients is to save you time & money, and give you recipes that not only taste delicious, but also will transform your body while giving you increased energy! If I was just interested in making money, I would be selling you a quick-fix, diet pill that lets you lose weight, but you would have numerous side effects and gain back all the weight within a month or two.

My program, backed by love and sincerity, is designed to give you a specific formula to lasting weight loss.

1.1 The Pillars

The science behind this results-driven program:

→ Time

Time is the commodity that we all want more of, and yet feel we most lack. We need to feel like we can adopt a program that adds to our quality of life, not take it away by requiring hours in the kitchen, hours in the gym, or hours in lethargy because we are eating so few calories. By shopping for simple five ingredient recipes, you save time at the grocery store.

When preparing meals with five ingredients, you save time in the kitchen. The majority of the 120+ recipes in this book take less than 15 minutes to make, and are prepared with fat-burning, whole foods that will transform your body when eating in proper proportions throughout the day, as directed by the accompanying meal plan guide.

→ Money

No more spending money on expensive shakes, diet pills or Dr. visits. These simple ingredients save you big money at the grocery store, and all the foods on the shopping list are "clean" foods, which translates into better health and fewer Dr. Visits.

Most "eat-clean" recipes have about 12 ingredients or more. Cooking with the **Eat, Drink and Shrink** recipes you will not skimp on taste and quality, but you will save money on your grocery bill. No more spending money on diet drinks, shakes or expensive weight loss meals. You will buy "real" food at your local grocery store.

→ Satisfying Foods

Most of us have tried programs where we were left unsatisfied - either the food was not filling, did not taste good, or no one else in the family could eat it. So after your program was over, you went back to your old habits and gained all the weight back.

The recipes in **Eat, Drink and Shrink** are designed for your whole family to enjoy, and will have you feeling satisfied so that you can make this way of eating your new lifestyle.

→ Shopping list

The foods on this program will literally transform your body! You will know exactly what foods to put in your kitchen to burn your stubborn body fat. The foods outlined in this program are all energy-driven foods, which means they allow you to eat more, have increased energy, all while dropping fat in all the right places!

→ Lasting Life Skills

In the **Eat, Drink and Shrink** plan, you will not only get a shopping list with all your recipes, but you will get chapters on how your mind works in sabotaging your success in weight loss. There are many great exercise and nutrition programs out there, but that is all they are—exercise and nutrition programs. There is a missing link in that equation and that is your mind.

Most of us are overweight because we are emotional eaters and those who sabotage themselves. There is a whole host of emotions going on that you need support on and understanding. You will get that support with this plan. You can read about how your mind works when it comes to weight loss or gain and how you can re-steer that in your life for the better.

You will also be able to join a community of "like-minded" individuals who are on the same path. You can receive support and love and weekly workouts to keep you motivated and on daily track with the **Forever Fit Challenge** Community!

→ Meal plan program

For free, you are going to get an accompany meal plan that works alongside the **Eat, Drink and Shrink** recipe book. This meal plan is not like any you have seen. It maps out your success so easily you will know exactly what to eat, in the right quantities, and percentages so you create the body of your dreams!

Not one person has tried this program and not seen results! It is in the science of the meal plan breakdown with success-driven recipes that will get you lasting results. No more being hungry, no more diet pills and drinks ever again! In addition, you are getting this **FREE** when you purchase the **Eat, Drink and Shrink** recipe book.

Chapter Two

Excuses

2.1 What compromises your efforts?

Through my own personal journey, as well as my work with thousands of coaching clients and seminar attendees over the last several years, I have noticed most sabotage is created because of the following seven reasons.

An article by, Sean Smith, breaks down the different ways we self-sabotage and how we can conquer it. I have included his article below:

> Virtually everyone sabotages his or her success to some degree. If you really want to find the underlying cause of the issue, you have to understand how and why the sabotaging habits are created in the first place.
>
> Then you can remove the cause, instead of doing what most people do their whole lives, which is chasing and trying to get rid of the symptoms.

All sabotage is self-created by the unconscious mind trying to keep us safe and comfortable.

I know it doesn't make much sense to think that our sabotaging habits were created for our own good, but it's true. The unconscious mind has one primary function that reigns supreme over all others – protecting and maintaining our physical and emotional safety, which includes being comfortable.

Therefore, if something external is perceived as a threat to our comfort or safety, our unconscious mind will step in to avoid the threat. It's like our internal defense system, and it's always on guard!

That's where sabotage is created. We develop habits – procrastination, perfectionism, disorganization, time management problems to keep us in our comfort zone, away from the potential harm.

But understand that's GREAT NEWS. Why? Because if you created your sabotage, then you, and only you, can *un-create* it, as long as you understand why you did it!

2.1.1 Scared of the Spotlight

When you achieve success, often a spotlight shines directly on you. This spotlight not only brightens your achievements, it can also shed light on any of your self-perceived limitations.

If you are unhappy with your physical appearance on any level, for example, being in the spotlight will probably intensify that displeasure. Why would you want to bring to light something that makes you unhappy, so others can ridicule you just as you constantly do to yourself?

Being in the spotlight also means you have greater visibility – and potential vulnerability. When you are in the spotlight, others may talk about you in a positive or negative way. You may shy away from the spotlight to avoid the increased potential for people to talk bad about you.

2.1.2 Greater Responsibility

This is one of the "Catch-22" factors of success. When you achieve your goals, you will likely have more responsibility – whether that is more people wanting you to mentor them, to inspire them. If you already feel you have enough or too much responsibility now, why would you want any more?

Another factor that often goes along with greater success is the increased pressure to stay on top. This is all a perception, and generally just pressure we put on ourselves – consciously or not. So the unconscious mind will generally do whatever it can to avoid that pressure and stay where we are … comfortable.

2.1.3 More Time Away from Family

Many people want to succeed so they can enjoy the freedom to spend more time with their family. However, if the path to success means spending more time away from family – working longer hours, taking more work home, increased traveling etc. you will have a values conflict.

Regardless of what goals you consciously want to achieve, your unconscious mind will never allow you to succeed if it means sacrificing time with your family, assuming that family time is one of your higher values. Now, some people might want to succeed so they can GET AWAY from their families, but that is a topic for a different book.

2.1.4 Greater Chance of Failing

Many of us do not have internal permission to even try to succeed, which is usually caused by the all-too-common fear of failure. The limiting belief here is that if you do not risk, you cannot fail. The reality, however, is if you do not risk, you will never succeed because you will not move beyond your current comfort zone.

If you are afraid to fail or have any notion that it is not okay to make mistakes, then your unconscious mind will do everything in its power to keep you right where you are – comfortable mediocrity. As crazy as it may sound, at the unconscious level, comfort is a higher priority than happiness!

2.1.5 Going to Lose Something You Enjoy

You might be sabotaging yourself if you already enjoy everything you are experiencing, and there are fears that you would lose something you currently have, if you were to increase your level of success. This stems from one of our most powerful fears – the fear of loss.

This is not an abundance mentality – it is actually very restrictive to believe that for every new thing that comes into your life, something else must go. Sometimes it certainly is the case, but not always. Do not let the either-or thinking hold you hostage. Ask, "How can I have both?" and let your mind find a way.

2.1.6 Fear of Connection

We all have abandonment issues to some degree, more than likely stemming from the earliest stages of our lives when we were literally dependent upon others to satisfy our basic survival needs. All it takes is one time for infants to cry and not get the attention they want to create the fear of abandonment.

In addition, if you have experienced any other form of emotional trauma – such as divorce, death of a loved one, abuse, etc., the abandonment issue is intensified. Either way, the unconscious mind believes the best way to avoid being abandoned by other people is to not allow yourself to get close to anyone. As long as you do not connect emotionally, you are safe.

In reality, however, physical and emotional connection is one of the most intense human desires. So keeping yourself "safe" by not connecting with people usually creates a bigger problem internally than the abandonment, if it were to happen. Sadly, lots of people use foods and their excess pounds as a refuge from all the pain and negative thoughts caused by breakups or by unshared love.

2.1.7 Fear of Judgment

This is a biggie because it applies to so many scenarios – talking to people you don't know, asking someone out on a date, speaking in public, networking, asking or answering questions, sales, recruiting, following up with clients, committing to your goals – the list is literally endless.

There are not many opportunities to succeed that do not involve the possibility of someone else's judgment. So if you are unconsciously committed to avoid being judged, you will forever be stuck.

The good news is that other people's judgments can only affect you if they match your own self-judgments. Therefore, when you clear up your feelings about yourself, nobody else's opinions have the power to control you.

2.2 How Can I Get Rid of These Conflicts

No matter what the reason causing the sabotage, the way around it is to prove to yourself that you can achieve success without the pain or sacrifice. Your unconscious mind does want you to succeed and to be happy, just not at the expense of your comfort and safety. Therefore, as soon as you remove the risk, you will have instant permission to succeed.

Removing that risk might involve releasing a limiting belief, letting go of emotional trauma from your past, erasing a fear, or just simply doing the thing you have been resisting and noticing the "bad" result did not happen. Regardless of what it entails, it is doable. In addition, more importantly – even if it takes a significant investment of your time, energy and money – do the work. You are worth it!

I believe to combat some of our excuses is to undergo a paradigm shift in our minds with our relation to food. A lot of us are stuck on the idea that foods high in fats & sugars are the best tasting. Yes, they taste good, but so does food high in good fats, proteins, and natural sugars. I am hoping that by trying out the recipes you will see eating clean can be a delicious and delightful experience!

Let us be honest, we eat the high sugared desserts and enjoy them in the moment, but afterwards, we don't feel so hot and we especially don't feel satisfied when we don't look and feel our best.

Why not change our paradigm and start telling ourselves we are not depriving ourselves by choosing foods from the snack section of the recipes? We can still honor our sweet tooth, but combine the urge for something sweet with the right combination of fats and natural sugars that will make us feel good afterwards.

We have rewarded ourselves with food our whole lives. As children our parents, teachers, grandparents were notorious at giving us reward with food. Food in our culture (actually in a lot of cultures), is used in other ways than to fuel our bodies. It is used for bonding time, to make us feel loved, and to celebrate or make us feel a sense of success.

I am reminded of this "reward for doing a great job" when my daughter comes home from school with a candy bar for getting 100% on her math test! Automatically she associates good behavior or excellence with a candy bar, (the wrong fat/sugar ratio you can get).

The above example is one of the reasons why so many of us (who are mothers), put our children to bed after a long, long day of tears, toddler defiance, cleaning up the home fifty plus times in one day, feel justified in sitting down to bowl of ice cream, or why we consume candy left over in the cupboard. It is in the recognition that we can begin to change our behaviors.

Does your body "really" want candy and ice cream after your long, hard day? Think about it. It wants a reward for handling all the work it has done whether at the office or juggling kids. It wants something that tastes good, but will give us the utmost energy, and something that will give us the extra boost of confidence in body, mind, and spirit.

In our recognition of our excuses and self-sabotage, we can start to implement the mental shift to resume eating clean, smaller portions at more frequent times throughout the day to feel, look and become our BEST selves!

Chapter Three

Knowledge is Power

3.1 Improving your eating habits

I remember the day I thought I was eating healthy. It was the day I had reduced fat wheat thins and was drinking soymilk instead of drinking regular whole milk.

After having 3 kids, training thousands of weight loss clients, I have discovered how wrong I was. Since then, I have discovered what foods actually aid in lasting weight loss, what foods create the most energy and health in your body and how to create the body of your dreams!

For those of you who have tried desperately to lose weight, either by deprivation or buying into the latest fads claiming low fat, low sugar, soy and are still not where you want your body to be ... *stay tuned.*

A simple rule that I follow: if it was naturally here on earth hundreds of years ago, and if our Paleolithic ancestors ate it, you most likely can eat it too. If it is chemically altered, processed, or refined, avoid it! Simple foods such as grass-fed, non-hormone meats, raw nuts and organically grown fruits and vegetables are always your best bet!

I would like to break it down in simple terms why this program works compared to the other thousands you have tried, or maybe saw results of, then despaired when you gained the weight back.

This program gives me great excitement because knowledge is power. It gives you the power to save time, the power to save money, and gives you the powerful feeling of seeing lasting RESULTS!

3.1.1 Why Do I Eat Only Certain Carbohydrates?

The carbs as outlined in the shopping list contain fewer sugars and have higher fiber content and less inflammatory response on the organs. Most grains we eat such as refined white breads, pastas, cereals, and quick oats and rice create inflammation in our organs due to the body trying to digest these processed grains or the gluten they contain (which ultimately can give you a distended gut).

3.1.2 Why is there a Protein Source in Each Meal?

Protein helps keep your blood sugar balanced. Protein takes longer to digest in the body, so you feel fuller (satiated) longer and it keeps your blood sugars down. This combination leads to a leaner, more energized body!

Eggs, fresh fish and meat (grass fed, free range) are some of the best ways to get protein in your body. Greek yogurt and Kefir (10-live cultures) have probiotics linked to fighting pathogens in your body and to decreasing inflammation in your organs.

Whey protein is a quick way to get protein, but you have to be careful. Many whey proteins contain lots of sugar or other chemicals. The whey I recommend is **BioTrust Low Carb**.

3.1.3 Why do I add Fat to Your Meal-Plan and Why Certain Fats?

Fats such as avocado, olive oil, grape seed oil, and raw unsalted nuts, have high amounts of HDL, which helps your body keep belly fat down, along with cholesterol. Fat is what keeps our organs 'slick,' our skin luminous and our hair shiny.

Consuming fats containing higher amounts of omega 3 and omega 6 in your day are highly recommended. We do not shop for canola oil/corn oil, or any other vegetable oil on the shopping list because it is so highly processed and chemically altered and contribute to stubborn body fat.

3.1.4 Why Do I Recommend You Take a Fish Oil Supplement?

Fish oil has healthy omega 3 fats and contains DHA and EPA. All of this is beneficial for your overall health, vitality, mental clarity, and the way your hair and skin look.

3.1.5 Why No Processed Sugar & Artificial Sweeteners in Meals?

Processed sugar is one of the worst things you can consume. After reading many scientific articles on the subject, I avoid it like the plague. It breaks down your cells and wreaks havoc on your organs (your skin especially, the largest organ).

Products containing high fructose corn syrup and refined sugar are processed sugars to avoid. This is one of the ingredients in many foods you think are healthy, foods like whole-wheat breads and yogurts.

There are other ways to get sweetness in your day by consuming fruits and raw, unaltered sugars, such as natural Stevia, honey, and 100% maple syrup. There is a lot of debate on whether raw sugar is any different from refined sugar.

They say "sugar is sugar". The way your body breaks down high fructose corn syrup and honey is completely different. Even though I do not discourage natural sugars, I recommend having small quantities, around 2 teaspoons per day. Many of us are addicted to sugar, hence the cravings for soft drinks, breads, condiments (especially ketchup), which are all loaded with sugar.

Follow the shopping list and the recipes 100% for two weeks. Riding your body of these substances will help subside your cravings and get your hormone levels back in alignment.

Artificial sweeteners do not contain calories, but that does not mean they are good for you, because these sweeteners are chemically altered. There are actual studies linking it to body fat with increased consumption. Some of the main artificial sweeteners are Splenda and Aspartame.

3.1.6 Why Organic, Fresh Foods Over Canned?

There is a lot of scientific evidence backing the harmful and addictive properties, but to make things simple, by eating fresh and organic you are limiting chemicals in your body, and getting the most nutrients per bite!

In addition, there is a link to fat and BPA. Canned foods and bottled drinks are notorious for containing both. The less processed, fabricated you can get your foods, the better you will be in meeting your wholesome, nutritional needs, and burning body fat.

3.1.7 Why Do I Encourage You to Consume Herbs & Spices?

Herbs and spices add flavor without added calories. Herbs and spices can have more nutritional value than a lot of our fruits and vegetables! Herbs and spices should be added to our foods whenever and as often as you can.

3.1.8 Why Coconut/Almond Milk Over Dairy Milk?

Despite trying to avoid getting rid of that phlegm feeling in your throat and creating unneeded coughing, there is a host of reasons to drink unsweetened almond and coconut milk over dairy. As you will notice, soymilk is not on the shopping list. Due to research, soymilk found at the grocery store amongst other soy products, is chemically altered & aids in creating belly fat.

Dairy milk is touted as a good supply of vitamin D and calcium, but there are many more nutrient dense ways to get calcium and vitamin D, without adding extra sugars (lactose), saturated fats, potential allergies, and cholesterol.

Daily exercise, daily sunlight, and consuming foods such

as almonds, spinach, kale and broccoli will give you adequate amounts of calcium and vitamin D.

3.1.9 Why Do I Have You Eating Every 2-3 Hours?

This is another huge factor in your success. When our body feels deprived, it slows down our metabolism. You have heard (or perhaps not), that skipping breakfast can be one of the worst ways to lose weight. When you awaken, your body needs the fuel to jump-start the fire (your metabolism). By eating, you are getting that little fire going, which burns up calories and gives your body energy.

Our bodies are efficient and have one purpose, unbelievably; it is not to look sexy. It is to have the most energy possible for everyday activities! By feeding your body, the key is every two to three hours; you are giving your body permission to burn up the previous meal for energy. Hence, by eating more frequently, you will feel more energized, increase your metabolism, and lean down at the same time!

3.1.10 Why The Specific Portions Amounts?

This is super important. I would like to take you through an analogy. Your stomach has a little fire inside, just a small, light burning fire, which is your metabolism. Have you heard the term "You have such a high metabolism you can eat all day long and never gain a pound"?

Have you ever wondered how the thin guy/girl can eat all day and still look GREAT? Well this is one of those keys. You too will be able to eat all day, drop weight, and look great. Our goal is to optimize weight loss and to maintain and increase energy. We want to keep the fire burning, not a raging bon fire or small burning embers, but at a steady rate.

When we eat the right amount of food in the right quantities, it is like putting a few logs on the fire. When we eat out, let us say a hamburger with fries, it is like creating a grease bonfire. When we skip meals or eat too little, that fire goes out which is the quickest way to hold on to fat?

3.1.11 Is Eating For Energy Better Than Eating For Weight Loss?

There is a host of reasons why I would rather eat for energy than eat for weight loss. Doesn't one sound more positive than the other? Our bodies need energy to serve and do all our daily activities.

Often in our quest for looking thin, having a simple paradigm shift in our minds creates a shift in our bodies as well. Focus on eating for fuel and energy & it takes out a whole lot of drama when you look at a bowl of ice cream versus a bowl of yogurt with fresh fruit.

3.1.12 Why and How to Eat Mindfully

This knowledge is powerful! Food was never meant to be shoveled in; hence, it wouldn't taste so darn good. I recommend taking a week to slow down your eating. Feel the texture of each bite; allow the many flavor combinations to explode in your mouth.

Take a minute to "feel" it, explore the texture of your food.

If you have a hard time with this exercise, one way to slow down your eating is to put your fork down between each bite. Doing this for a week will help you slow down and "taste" your food.

When you are mindful and enjoy each bite, you will eat less, you will feel more satisfied, and if you are eating emotional, it will bring you back to the moment of why you are eating. You are eating to fuel your body. You are eating to increase your energy. You are eating for the enjoyment of food.

3.2 Joining the Forever Fit Challenge Community is Critical

I have been a trainer working with individuals for years! Even though I see results with all compliant clients, I have noticed the ones who cannot afford lifelong training with me, find it very difficult to keep the results. This is not because they do not have the tools or the will.

Human nature needs to feel like they belong, as if they have a support system & a place where they can resonate with "like minded" people. Being a part of the community is vital to everyone's long-term success. For those of you who may be recovering alcoholics, you know this all too well.

When you have had abuse with alcohol, it is best to build relations with people who do not drink. Not all of you have abuse with food, yet, many of you do! This community will inspire you daily to keep motivated. You will gain a sense of belonging. You will be in a community to pick you up on your bad days.

It is in the community that it all comes together. New weekly workout videos from Danette, monthly telecals with Danette, weekly motivational articles on the power of your mind, new flavorful recipes that are quick and easy, and a place to ask questions and receive answers will help you and keep you living your most abundant life. Even I need a community of likeminded health people to keep me on track. You can access the Forever Fit Site at **theforeverfitchallenge.com/monthly/.**

I am inspired and encouraged each day to make healthy choices and to pass it on to my children!

Chapter Four

Water and Fat Loss

I want to educate you on some of the many benefits of water because I think we forget how very important it is to us reaching our goals!

Your goal is to consume ¾ to 1 gallon per day, to not only flush fat and aid in weight loss, but to flush toxins from your body.

Did you know that not drinking enough plain water is as harmful to your heart as smoking? While not as glamorous, the degree of benefit from plain water reportedly surpasses drinking moderate amounts of wine, taking aspirin and other preventive measures.

Drinking five glasses of water daily can decrease the risk of colon cancer by up to 45%, can slash the risk of breast cancer by up to 79%, and can reduce the risk of bladder cancer by up to 50%. Preliminary research indicates that 8-10 glasses of water a day could significantly ease back pain and joint pain for up to 80% of sufferers.

- Lack of water is the number one trigger for daytime fatigue.

- A mere 2% drop in body water can trigger fuzzy short-term memory, trouble with basic math, and difficulty focusing on the computer screen.

- In 37% of Americans, the body's thirst mechanism is so weak that it is often mistaken for hunger.

- One glass of water shut down midnight hunger pangs for almost 100% of the dieters in a University of Washington study.

- Last but not certainly least: mild dehydration will slow down one's metabolism as much as 3%.

Chapter Five

Herbs

5.1 The natural taste enhancers

Herbs have been in use for thousands of years to flavor and preserve food, treat ailments, ward off pests and diseases, as an air freshener, as a decorative addition to our homes, offices, and as an overall enhancer in our lives.

The herbs I am going to list are ones I recommend you have in your home for many reasons. This nutrition book is about being thin around your waistline and it is about saving time and money. These herbs are in line with the program and accomplish the task.

Many of the recipes in the book contain the herbs listed below. Additionally, there is something satisfying about picking food or herbs from the herb plants in your home and adding them directly to your recipes. You can have as many herbs as you want.

I recommend having as many as is joyful for you, but for simple purposes I am going to list five. These herbs help with digestion, fat loss and the overall beauty of your skin. Herbs are great for flavoring your foods without adding many calories --major plus.

You can always buy these herbs at your local supermarket, but if you want something simple and want to save money then I will tell you exactly what to buy, where you can buy them and how to take care of them. If you have herbs in your home and on hand, it saves time driving to the grocery store, saves time thinking about herb choices and of course, saves more on overall cost.

5.1.1 Sweet Basil

Benefits: Sweet Basil known more for its pleasant taste than for its medicinal effects on our bodies, due to its mild sedative properties, herbalists traditionally prescribed basil as a tea for easing nervous irritability.

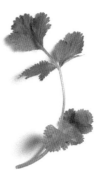

Buy: At most major distributors of plants. Walmart carries it.

Care: Water every day and allow sunlight daily. You can also pull off leaves and add them to any dish for an Italian flavor. You can mix basil in a good olive oil, allow the flavor to seep into the oil, and add a small amount of basil oil to pizzas and add to salads (see recipes listed in this book).

5.1.2 Aromatic Basil Oil

Delicious, use on salads, meats etc.; take a jar and layer basil leaves in the bottom of the jar and sprinkle each layer with sea salt. Then at the top add a good quality olive oil. Seal the jar securely and store in the refrigerator. Allow several days for the oil to infuse with the flavor of the basil. Use the leaves and the oil for seasoning.

5.1.3 Cilantro

I absolutely love this plant and its flavor. It spices most dishes to perfection.

Benefits: Also known more for its taste, but of course contains antioxidants.

Buy: Any major plant distributor. Buy and repot.

Care: Water every day and needs daily sunlight.

5.1.4 Lemon Balm

Lemon balm is very similar to mint, but takes on a lemony flavor. It complements most foods. You can add it to tea, salads, fruit dishes, and chilled summer drinks.

Benefits: Lemon Balm acts as a mild sedative and has mood-enhancing effects, commonly used to treat sleep disorders, restlessness, anxiety, and depression.

Buy: Buy from all major distributors.

Care: Care by providing water and daily sunlight.

5.1.5 Mint

You can buy mint in many different ranges. Pick the one that tastes best to you. Mint is great for teas.

Benefits: Peppermint produces notable relaxing effects on the gut and can help to relive indigestion, nausea, gas, and cramping. Many clinical trials have verified a therapeutic effect of the herb on many of the symptoms of irritable bowel syndrome, including diarrhea, constipation, bloating and abdominal pain.

Buy: Buy from most major distributors.

Care: Water and provide daily sunlight.

5.1.6 Rosemary

Few herbs are universally grown & loved as much as rosemary. This herb is great on most chicken/fish/meat dishes.

Benefits: The main benefits or this herb is combating general fatigue & depression and for improving poor circulation.

Buy: Purchase from most distributors.

Care: Water and expose to sunlight daily.

Chapter Six

Shopping List & Exchange List

6.1 Shopping List

"What you put in your mouth is 80% of the way you are going to look and feel"

6.1.1 Protein

- Chicken
- Turkey
- Extra lean ground turkey
- Lean hambu
- Lean steak
- Beef filet
- Tilapia
- Buffalo
- Tuna
- Egg whites
- Whole eggs
- Haddock
- Cold or any white fish
- Shrimp
- Scallops
- Bison
- Cottage cheese – look for one without a lot of fillers and added ingredients
- **Whey Protein powder**
- Egg white protein powder

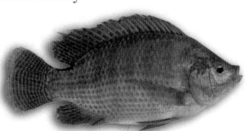

TILAPIA

- Lobster
- Venison
- Plain Greek yogurt
- Kefir
- Chia seeds
- Hemp seeds

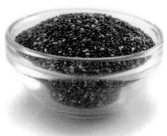

6.1.2 Carbohydrates

- Slow cooked oatmeal – you can buy gluten free if you are sensitive to gluten
- Lentils
- Beans (kidney, red, black, cannelloni)
- Sweet potatoes
- White potatoes
- Red potatoes
- Quinoa
- Millet
- Amaranth
- Buckwheat
- Slow cooked brown rice
- Pumpkin
- Ezckicl brcad (may contain gluten)
- Hummus (preferably homemade)

QUINOA

*Most rices and grains come in flour form at the grocery store for baking

Good flours to use for baking pancakes, muffins, waffles, and other desserts are: coconut flour, buckwheat flour, spelt flour, brown rice flour, and almond meal/flour.

6.1.3 Fruits and Veggies

All are acceptable, but go for variety and lots of color.

6.1.4 Good fats

- Flax oil
- Pecans (all nuts consumed raw and unsalted)
- Olive oil
- Almonds
- Walnuts
- Raw/natural peanut butter
- Raw/natural almond butter
- Avocado
- Coconut oil
- Grape seed oil
- Olives
- Hummus

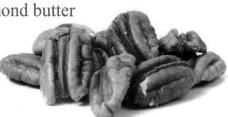

PECANS

6.1.5 Condiments

All herbs and spices

- Mustard
- Chili peppers
- Chives
- Cilantro
- Dill
- Ginger
- Garlic
- Lemon verbena
- Mint
- Orange mint
- Oregano

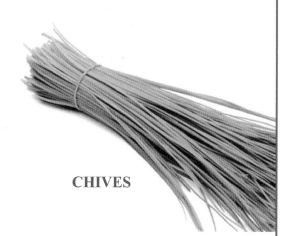

CHIVES

- Parsley
- Rosemary
- Sweet basil
- Tarragon
- Thyme
- Turmeric

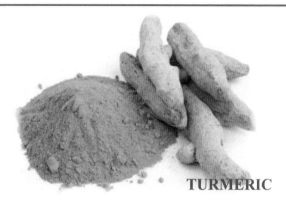

TURMERIC

The above lists of herbs are the ones I like using when I cook. They also have many healing proponents and considered FREE FOODS!

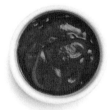

NOTE: If you are someone who has to have ketchup on everything, find ketchup that uses maple syrup, honey or Stevia in it, as opposed to high fructose corn syrup. Always use sparingly.

6.1.6 Random Foods

- Almond milk
- Coconut milk
- Rice milk
- Stevia for sweetener
- Honey
- Maple syrup (100%)
- Ground flax seed
- Teas (try to choose mainly decaffeinated)
- Mushrooms (free food)
- 100% raw cocoa powder
- Unsweetened coconut flakes

6.1.7 Multivitamins

- **Multivitamins**
- **Fish oil** (must be USP certified or pharmaceutical grade quality)

6.1.8 Fluids

- Drink ¾ of a gallon to a gallon of water per day

6.1.9 Foods to Avoid

- Diet soda
- Carbonated drinks
- Creamy based salad dressings
- Deli meats
- Processed soy products
- Alcohol
- Cheesy products
- Frozen food dinners
- Cream in coffee (use almond or coconut milk)
- Artificial sweeteners

6.2 Food Exchanges

This book is a compilation of my research. I am putting the foods in the categories I do for a purpose in helping you lose fat efficiently, while providing your body with the adequate amounts of vitamins and nutrients it needs each day. Each one of my recipes breaks down the percentages in each recipe.

Of course these are not exact measurements (I am not an exact kind of person), but the cool thing is, it works! I have tried this on 100's of people and have seen them drop weight. The science lies in the foods chosen, the portion amounts, and takes into account the time of delivery into your system.

The science behind 5 ingredients or less recipes is to save you time, money, and calories, using only clean, nutrient dense food options—hence limiting most of our excuses.

6.2.1 Free Foods

These foods can be eaten as often as you would like:

*mustard	*mushrooms
*herbs	*herbal tea
*spices	*water
*lemons and limes	

Chapter 5 is about herbs. I would recommend growing and having them in your home. Herbs are inexpensive, easy to use, give you bountiful flavors, and you can place pots of herbs on your window-seal, herbs like, basil, cilantro, rosemary, dill, and mint.

6.2.2 Food Exchanges

NOTE: You can use this to exchange certain foods in the recipes that you may not love for foods that you do love. This will give you an idea of how much of what food you can exchange to stay in correct portions of fats, proteins, veggies, fruits, and carbs.

Carbs:

½ cup carb {
½ gluten free pita
1 tortilla size pizza crust recipe
1 slice Ezekiel bread (whole grain bread product) or 1 slice gluten
free whole grain bread
½ cup cooked oatmeal, all variety rice, amaranth, beans
¼ cup hummus (hummus will also be added as a fat)

Fats:

1 tbsp. fat {
1 handful of raw unsalted nuts (approx. 1/8 cup)
1 tbsp. almond/peanut butter
1 tbsp. oil
½ avocado
1 tbsp. hummus
4 Edamame shells or 1/8 cup

Veggies / fruits = I am totaling them in their raw uncooked form.

Proteins:

3 oz. {
approximately one deck of cards worth of meat
1 scoop of whey protein
½ cup of cottage cheese, kefir or Greek yogurt
3 egg whites or 2 whole eggs

NOTE: I would go sparingly on the sugars and milks, 2 tsp. /day on sugars and 1/8-1/4 cup of almond/coconut milk/day.

In addition, if the recipe is in the snack area, do not eat it for dinner or lunch, as those items tend to have more sugars in them and you will go over your limit for the day. Recipes should stay within their categories.

Chapter Seven

Eat, Drink, and Shrink Recipes

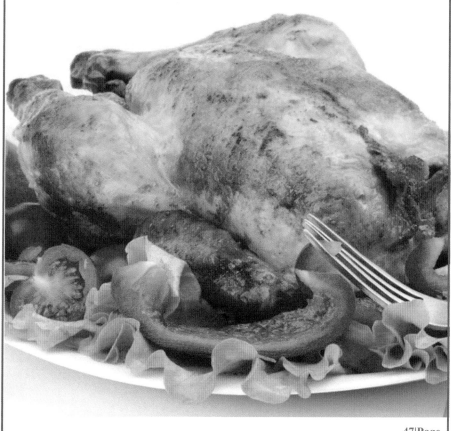

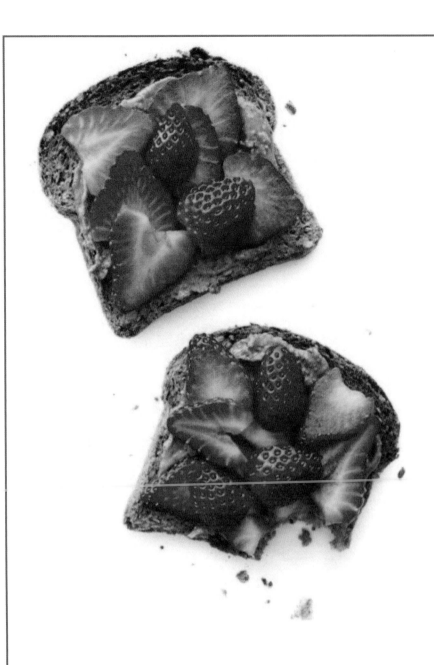

BREAKFAST

Oatmeal & Hot Cereals

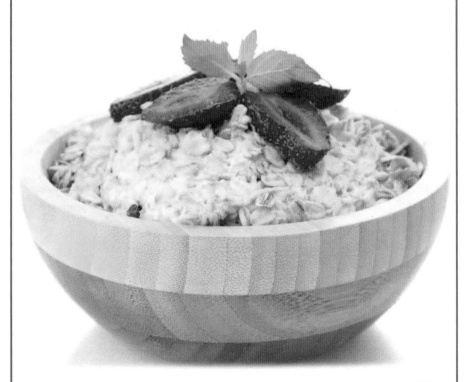

7.1 Oatmeal & Hot Cereals

Buckwheat, oatmeal and eggs are a staple in my home for breakfast. I think some of us have an aversion to oatmeal because it brings back memories when we were younger and our mom placed bland tasting, mushy oatmeal in front of us, and a large quantity to boot.
By the fourth bite, we were textured out and completely grossed out. My kids love oatmeal and that is because I try to add a little spice & variety.

7.1.1 SIMPLE BUCKWHEAT/QUINOA/OATMEAL PREPERATION

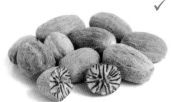

- ✓ Take ¼ cup oats/buckwheat/quinoa
- ✓ Cook with ½ cup water in microwave for 50 seconds
- ✓ Top with ¼ cup of your choice of fruit

Once you have chosen your fruit, pick your nuts and spices accordingly.

NOTE: I am not kidding; your oatmeal may start tasting like cobbler. The idea is to get creative and see what sizzles your taste buds. Remember to stay within the percentage of fruits and fats you need. It truly is delicious!

SPICE SUGGESTIONS FOR OATMEAL

- Cinnamon
- Nutmeg
- Cardommon

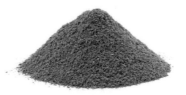

GREAT COMBINATIONS FOR OATMEAL

- ✓ Coconut/banana/walnuts
- ✓ Berries/pecans or almonds
- ✓ Peaches/walnuts
- ✓ Raisins/walnuts/bananas
- ✓ Cranberries/walnuts
- ✓ Bananas/sunflower seeds/peanut butter

NOTE: If you like your oatmeal creamy instead of thick, I add ¼ cup of almond or coconut milk. For a little added sweetness I add 1 tsp. Stevia, 1 tsp. maple syrup or 1 tsp. honey.

7.1.2 CHOCOLATE OATMEAL/BUCKWHEAT/ QUINOA

Nutritional Information: *(½ cup carbs, 1 tbsp. fat, ¼-½ cup fruit)*

- ✓ ½ cup oats/buckwheat/quinoa (approx. ¼ cup dry oats with 1/2 cup water added) then cooked
- ✓ 1/4 cup unsweetened almond milk/coconut milk
- ✓ 2 tbsp. dark chocolate chips

NOTE: If you are trying to lose weight or trying to lose the last 10 pounds, take out the chocolate chips and add 1 tsp. Stevia & add ½ tsp. of cocoa powder.

To add a protein source, you can add 1 scoop of chocolate whey protein or you can add 3 oz. Greek yogurt or eggs to the side. You can top oatmeal with ¼-½ cup cherries, berries, or bananas.

7.1.3 BANANA WALNUT OATMEAL/BUCKWHEAT/QUINOA

Nutritional Information: *(½ cup carbs, 1 tbsp. fat, ¼ cup fruit)*

- ✓ ¼ cup dry oats/buckwheat/quinoa cooked with
- ✓ ½ cup water in microwave for approx. 55 seconds
- ✓ 1/8 cup walnuts
- ✓ ¼ cup sliced banana
- ✓ 1 tsp. Stevia for sweetness

7.1.4 SUPERPOWER MUESLI

Nutritional Information: ½ cup = *(3 oz. protein, ¼ cup carbs, ¼ cup fruit)*

Takes 10 minutes to prepare and then refrigerate at least 8 hrs.

- ✓ 2 ½ cup plain Greek yogurt
- ✓ 1 ½ cup old-fashioned rolled oats
- ✓ ¼ cup raisins
- ✓ 2 tsp. orange zest grated
- ✓ ¼ tsp. nutmeg

Mix and then refrigerate.
Take ½ cup and top with ¼ cup of fresh fruits.

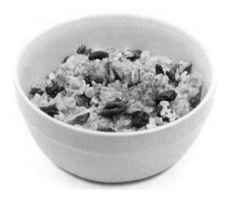

7.1.5 MAPLE-PECAN QUINOA

Nutritional Information: *(½ cup carbs, 1 tbsp. fat, ½ cup fruit) To add 2-3 oz. protein to your meal add 2 boiled eggs or ½ cup fat-free Greek yogurt*

- ✓ 1/4 cup quinoa mixed with
- ✓ 1/4cup almond/ rice/ coconut milk and 1/4 cup water
- ✓ 1/4 tsp. vanilla extract
- ✓ 2 tbsp. chopped pecans
- ✓ 1/2 cup fresh or frozen berries

Cook ¼ cup quinoa with ¼ cup almond/rice/coconut milk and ¼ cup water. Top with ¼ tsp. vanilla extract, 1 tsp. 100% maple syrup, 2 tbsp. chopped pecans, & ½ cup fresh or frozen berries. If you need some sweetness add 1 tbsp. 100% maple syrup

7.1.6 BUCKWHEAT CEREAL

Nutritional Information: *(½ cup carbs, ½ Tbsp. fat, ¼ cup fruit)*

- ✓ 2/3 cup water
- ✓ 1/3 cup uncooked buckwheat
- ✓ 1/2 banana or fruit of choice
- ✓ 1 tbsp. crushed walnuts or nut of choice

Microwave for 4 minutes, then top buckwheat with 1/2 banana, 1 tsp. honey (optional) and 1 tbsp. of crushed walnuts.

Quinoa Fun Facts: It is a seed, not a grain. It is a complete protein. It is loaded with fiber, Iron, magnesium. and cooks just like rice.

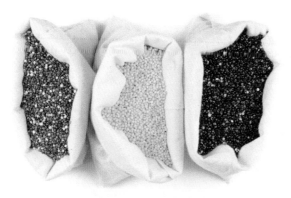

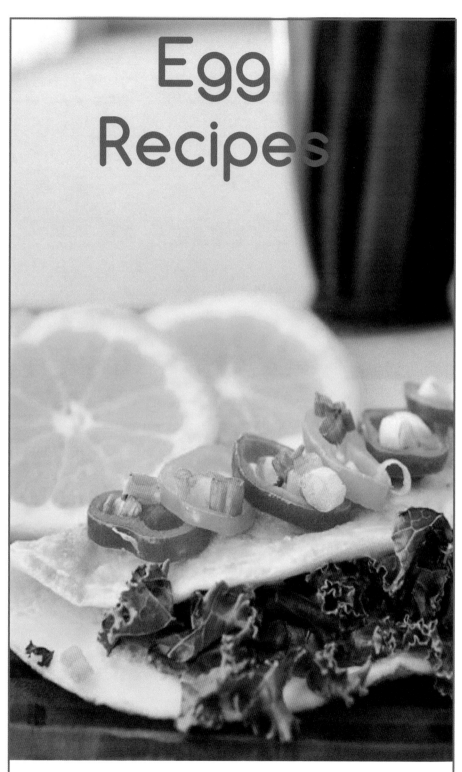

Egg
Recipes

7.2 Egg Recipes

Eggs are one of the simplest and best ways to get protein in the morning. There are so many health benefits to the egg and once again, you can create masterpieces with the egg and different veggies/lean meats and salsas. If I am not having boiled eggs, I tend to make scrambled eggs just because of the simplicity of it.

If you want something fancier, you can scramble your eggs before placing them in the skillet to make an omelet. You can also add a verity of chopped veggies, garlic, onion, curry powder, or salsas (mango, etc.).

By cooking three eggs and adding ¼-½ cup chopped veggies of choice and sprinkling curry powder on it, I have made sure I have my veggies and protein to start my day. If you want to add a healthy fat, you can always top with avocado, feta, or hummus.

7.2.1 EGGS & TOAST

Nutritional Information: (*3 oz. protein, ½ cup carbs, ¼ cup fruit*)

- ✓ 2 eggs
- ✓ 1 slc. Ezekiel bread
- ✓ 1/2 grapefruit

Cook 2 eggs, either well or with some runny yolk (whichever way you like it). Place on top of 1 slice toasted Ezekiel bread, sprinkle of sea salt (minimally) and pepper to taste.

7.2.2 BACON & EGG WITH TOAST

Nutritional Information: (½ carbs, 3 oz. protein, ½ cup veggies)

- ✓ 2 slices of turkey bacon cooked
- ✓ 1 egg scrambled
- ✓ Toast 1 slice of Ezekiel bread
- ✓ 1 tomato sliced

You can either eat individually and or stack on top of your toast.

7.2.3 SOFT BOILED EGG SALAD

Nutritional Information: *(2-3 oz. protein, ¼ cup veggies, 1 Tbsp. fat)*

- ✓ ¼ cup arugula
- ✓ 1 tbsp. goat cheese
- ✓ 2 soft boiled eggs
- ✓ Handful of shredded basil

Toss with 1 tbsp. good quality balsamic vinegar. Place 2 soft-boiled eggs on top

NOTE: Cooking tip on the soft-boiled eggs, boil them for 9 minutes, take out immediately, and run cold water over them and then peel. Pick a carb preference from the exchange list, ex. oats or Ezekiel toast with a side of fruit or topped with fruit.

7.2.4 SPINACH SCRAMBLE

Nutritional Information: *(3 oz. protein, ½ cup veggies)*

- ✓ 3 eggs or 2 eggs and 1 egg white
- ✓ 1/2 cup spinach
- ✓ 2 tbsp. chopped onion

Place spinach & onion in skillet, cook until spinach wilts, add eggs and scramble until fully cooked. To add a fat, top with ½ an avocado (1 Tbsp. fat) or 1 Tbsp. feta cheese (1 Tbsp. fat)

NOTE: Pick a carb preference from the exchange list, ex. oats or Ezekiel toast or ¼ cup fruit to the side.

7.2.5 TOAST WITH EGG & TOMATO

Nutritional Information: *(½ cup carbs, 3 oz. protein, ½ cup veggies)*

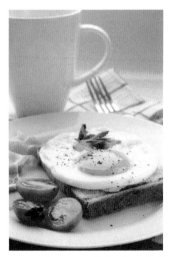

- ✓ 2 eggs cooked
- ✓ Toast 1 slice Ezekiel bread
- ✓ 1 tomato sliced
- ✓ fresh basil
- ✓ balsamic vinaigrette

Stack all ingredients on top of toast and top with fresh basil and drizzle on balsamic vinaigrette.

7.2.6 RANCHERO BURRITO

Nutritional Information: *(3 oz. protein, ½ cup veggies, ½ cup carbs)*

- ✓ 2 eggs
- ✓ ¼ cup cottage cheese
- ✓ ½ cup chopped veggies of choice (tomatoes, green pepper and onion are good)
- ✓ ¼ cup black beans
- ✓ Handful of cilantro and red pepper flakes to taste

In a skillet, combine eggs, cottage cheese, veggies, and beans. Cook and stir together. Once cooked, place in a bowl and eat.

7.2.7 TOMATO, ARTICHOKE & FETA FRITTATA

Nutritional Information: *(3 oz. protein, ½ cup veggies, 1 Tbsp. fat)*

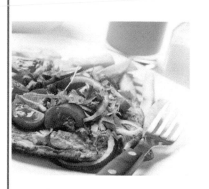

- ✓ 1 egg and 2 egg whites (whisked together)
- ✓ 1/ 4 cup chopped tomato
- ✓ ¼ cup canned artichoke hearts drained and chopped
- ✓ 1 tsp. chopped shallot

Cook artichoke, shallots, and tomato for 2 minutes and then add egg mixture. Then cook until eggs are firm. Top with 1 tbsp. feta (optional fat).

Optional: top with fresh cilantro.

NOTE: Pick a carb preference from the exchange list, ex. oats or Ezekiel toast with a side of fruit or topped with fruit.

7.2.8 WARM EGG WHITE/SPINACH QUICHE

Nutritional Information: *(½ cup = 3 oz. protein, ½ cup veggies, ½ Tbsp. fat)*

- ✓ add 6 egg whites
- ✓ ½ red onion chopped
- ✓ 8 oz. spinach around 2 ½ cup fresh
- ✓ 2 gloves of garlic chopped fine (sauté in skillet)
- ✓ ¼ cup feta cheese or ½ cup ricotta

Sauté in skillet garlic, onion and spinach. After spinach is wilted (approx. 2 min.), add whisked eggs & cheese to mixture. Mix and bake at 350-degrees for 30 minutes.

Optional: Top with fresh cilantro.

NOTE: You can replace the 6 egg whites for 5 whole eggs if you prefer.

> Eggs Fun Facts: Scrambled, poached, or hard boiled, eggs keep your blood sugar steady and provide many of the vitamins and minerals you need.

7.2.9 SOUTHWESTERN SCRAMBLE

Nutritional Information: *(3 oz. protein, ½ cup veggies, ¼ cup carbs)*

- ✓ 3 eggs
- ✓ ½ tomato diced
- ✓ ¼ cup onion diced
- ✓ ¼ cup refried beans or black beans
- ✓ ½ cup spinach

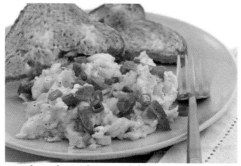

Add onion and spinach to skillet and cook until spinach is wilted. Add whisked eggs, beans and tomatoes. Cook until eggs are done. Top with ½ avocado (optional); add 1 tbsp. fat, total (if you add this) and top with fresh cilantro to taste.

Waffles /
Pancakes /
Crepes

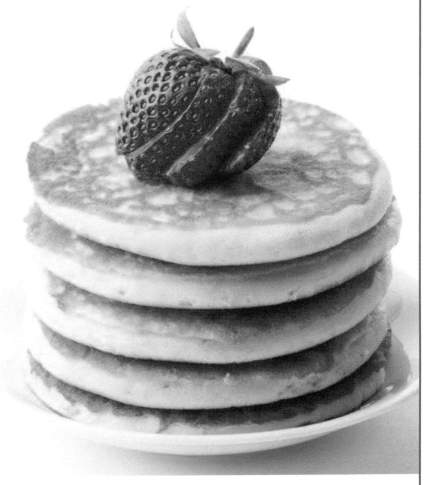

7.3 Waffles / Pancakes / Crepes

7.3.1 FILLING PROTEIN PANCAKES

Nutritional Information: *(4 oz. protein, ¼ cup fruit, 1/8 cup carbs-very minimal)*

Makes 1 large pancake

- ✓ Mix together 2 egg whites
- ✓ 1 scoop vanilla whey protein
- ✓ 3 tbsp. slow cooked oats
- ✓ Half-mashed banana
- ✓ 1 tsp. cinnamon
  2 tbsp. water

Heat skillet and pour on mixed mixture, cook until lightly brown on both sides. Top with 1 tsp. 100% maple syrup or eat plan. Delicious!

7.3.2 BANANA COCONUT CREPES

Nutritional Information: *(1 crepe = 3 oz protein, ½ tbsp. fat, ½ cup carbs, ¼-½ cup fruit (depending on how much fruit you put on your crepe and how much you eat)*

Makes 2 crepes

- ✓ 5 eggs (3 whole, 2 egg whites)
- ✓ 1 cup lite coconut milk
- ✓ 1 cup buckwheat flour (you can use any flour you prefer, spelt, brown rice flour etc). I chose buckwheat because it is a superfood
- ✓ sliced banana

Mix and pour a thin layer into skillet, once almost cooked, slice bananas and put unsweetened coconut flakes (optional) in, fold in half, cook fully.

Top with any favorite toppings as long as it is pure/natural/clean. I love adding 1 tbsp. fat free Greek yogurt and 1 tsp. 100% maple syrup.

7.3.3 HEARTY FRENCH TOAST

Nutritional Information: *(2 oz. protein, ½ cup carbs, ¼ cup fruit, ½ tsp. fat)*

- ✓ 2 eggs
- ✓ 1 slice Ezekiel bread
- ✓ 1 tsp. vanilla
- ✓ 2 tsp. cinnamon

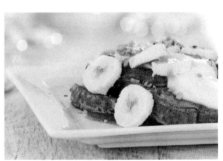

Mix & whip together 2 eggs, 1 tsp. vanilla/ 2 tsp. cinnamon. Heat skillet and cover the bread of choice in egg mixture, and cook on medium heat for approximately 30 seconds on each side.

Top with 1/2 sliced banana and 1 tbsp. walnuts, 1 tsp. 100% maple syrup. Top with ¼ cup Greek yogurt to add 1 oz. protein if you like. This is yummy and so good for you too.

NOTE: Egg Mixture is enough for 2 slc. of Ezekiel bread

7.3.4 CHOCOLATE POWER WAFFLES

Nutritional Information: *(1 pancake or waffle = 2 oz. protein, ¼ cup carbs, ¼ cup veggies, ¼ cup fruit if add fruit to top)*

Makes 4 small waffles

In blender or mixer, add:

- ✓ 2 scoops of chocolate whey protein
- ✓ 2 scoops of chocolate amazing grass (optional, but what a great way to get all your Superfoods)
- ✓ 2 eggs
- ✓ ½ cup oats/buckwheat flour or flour of choice from the shopping list
- ✓ 1 tsp. baking powder (optional)
  1 cup water

Place mixture on hot griddle for pancakes or on a hot waffle maker for waffles.

NOTE: I top these with fresh sliced bananas and 1 tsp. maple syrup. Yum!

7.3.5 BLUEBERRY PANCAKES

Nutritional Information: *(2 small sized pancakes = 2 oz. protein, ¼ cup carbs, ¼ cup fruit).*

Makes 4 small pancakes

In blender combine:

- ✓ 1 cup slow cooked oats
- ✓ 1/2 cup cottage cheese
- ✓ 2 eggs
- ✓ blueberries
- ✓ 1 tsp. vanilla

Blend than stir in 1 cup blueberries; eat 2 pancakes with 1 Tsp. 100% maple syrup.

7.3.6 SUNDAY MORNING PANCAKES

Nutritional Information: *(1 pancake= 2 oz. protein, 1/3 cup carbs, and ¼ cup fruit).* This is a perfect, slimming recipe

Makes 2 pancakes

- ✓ 3/4 cup oatmeal ground up in blender
- ✓ 2 egg whites
- ✓ 1 tsp. cinnamon
- ✓ 1 tsp. flax seed (grounded)
- ✓ 1/4 cup banana slices
  ½ cup water

Blend all together, pour in hot pan (slice ¼ cup banana slices on top of batter). Cook on both sides until lightly brown, approx. 1-2 minutes on medium heat. Enjoy!

7.3.7 FLAVORFUL PUMPKIN WAFFLES

Nutritional Information: 1 waffle = *(2 oz. protein, ½ cup carbs, ¼ cup fruit), if you top with fruit, add that amount to your fruit total.* Top with ¼ cup Greek yogurt to add 1 oz. protein if you like.

Makes 3-4 waffles

- ✓ 1 1/2 cup brown rice flour, buckwheat, almond or spelt flour
- ✓ 2 eggs
- ✓ 1 cup pumpkin puree
- ✓ 1/4 cup applesauce
- ✓ 1 tbsp. pumpkin pie spice
  1 2/3 cup water

Mix ingredients together in your blender, pour over your waffle iron, and cook through. Top with 100% maple syrup or your favorite fruit.

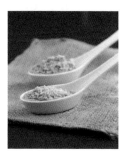

BROWN RICE AND BUCKWHEAT FLOUR

Buckwheat, amaranth, coconut, almond, and brown rice flours are a great substitute to our favorite breakfast meals without compromising taste and our waistline.

Muffins

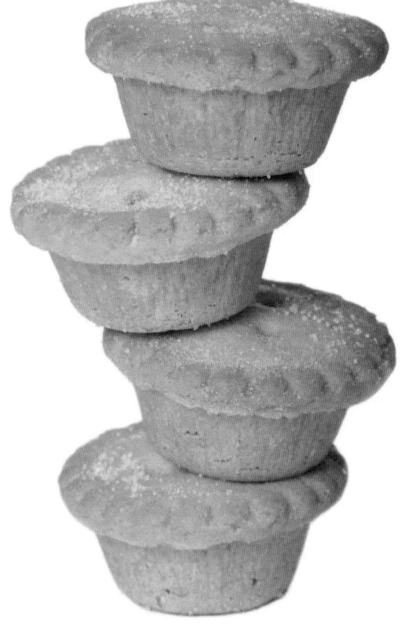

7.4 Muffins

Who says muffins cannot be nutritious and delicious. What I love about muffins is their resemblance to cupcakes. My family loves these.

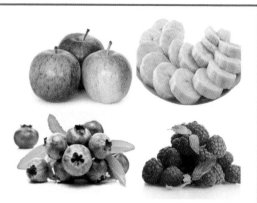

7.4.1 FLUFFY PROTEIN MUFFINS

Nutritional Information: (*2 muffins = 3 oz. protein, ½ cup carbs, ¼ cup fruit*)

Makes 16 muffins

- ✓ 4 eggs
- ✓ 2 cups oats blended into a powder
- ✓ 1 cup unsweetened applesauce
- ✓ 1/3 cup cottage cheese
- ✓ ½ cup whey protein powder
- ✓ 1 tbsp. vanilla extract

Pre-heat oven to 350-degrees, and pour ingredients into a blender and blend until smooth. You can make any flavored muffin you want by mixing in (by hand) any fruit you desire, by adding approx. 1/2 c.-1 c. of fruit to the recipe. Pour into greased w. coconut oil muffin tin or use silicone or tin muffin cups.

Cook until toothpick comes out clean (about 40 minutes).

7.4.2 CHOCOLATE BANANA MUFFINS

- ✓ 4 eggs
- ✓ 2 cups oats blended into a powder
- ✓ 1 cup unsweetened applesauce
- ✓ 1/3 cup cottage cheese
- ✓ ½ cup whey protein powder
- ✓ 1 tbsp. vanilla extract
- ✓ ½ cup sliced banana
- ✓ 1 tbsp. unsweetened cocoa powder

Use chocolate flavored whey protein powder

7.4.3 FAT BURNING BLUEBERRY MUFFINS

Nutritional Information: (*2 muffins = 3 oz. protein, 1 tbsp. fat, ¼ cup fruit*)

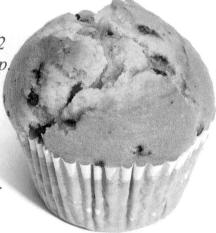

Makes 8-10 muffins

- ✓ 3 eggs
- ✓ 1 cup almond butter
- ✓ 1 cup almond meal/almond flour
- ✓ ½ cup raw honey
- ✓ ½ cup fresh/frozen blueberries or any fruit you want
- ✓ 1/3 cup unsweetened shredded coconut
- ✓ 1/3 cup Virgin Coconut Oil, melted
- ✓ ½ tsp. baking soda
- ✓ ½ tsp. baking powder
- ✓ ¼ tsp. sea salt

✓ Pinch of cinnamon

Preheat your oven to 350 degrees. Mix all ingredients together. Line muffin tin with tin muffin cups or silicone muffin cups. Place ingredients in muffin cups and bake approx.. 15-20 min.

7.4.4 APPLE CINNAMON MUFFINS
Nutritional Information: (*2 muffins = 3 oz. protein, 1 tbsp. fat, ¼ cup fruit*)

Makes 8-10 muffins

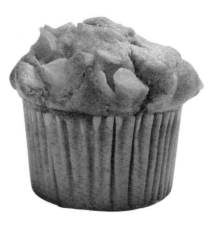

✓ 3 eggs
✓ 1 cup almond butter
✓ 1 cup almond meal/almond flour
✓ ½ cup raw honey
✓ 1/3 cup Virgin Coconut Oil, melted
✓ ½ tsp. baking soda
✓ ½ tsp. baking powder
✓ ¼ tsp. sea salt
✓ 1 tsp. of cinnamon
✓ 1/2 cup fresh chopped apples

Preheat your oven to 350 degrees. Mix all ingredients together. Line muffin tin with tin muffin cups or silicone muffin cups. Place ingredients in muffin cups and bake for approx. 15-20 min.

7.4.5 BANANA NUT MUFFINS

Nutritional Information: (*2 muffins = 3 oz. protein, 1 tbsp. fat, ¼ cup fruit*)

Makes 8-10 muffins

- ✓ 3 eggs
- ✓ 1 cup almond butter
- ✓ 1 cup almond meal/almond flour
- ✓ ½ cup raw honey
- ✓ 1/3 cup Virgin Coconut Oil, melted
- ✓ 1 banana, mashed in with all the ingredients
- ✓ ½ tsp. baking soda
- ✓ ½ tsp. baking powder
- ✓ ¼ tsp. sea salt
- ✓ Pinch of cinnamon
- ✓ ¼ cup crushed walnuts (or raw unsalted nut of choice), stirred in to mixture at the end.

Preheat your oven to 350 degrees. Mix all ingredients together. Line muffin tin with tin muffin cups or silicone muffin cups. Place ingredients in muffin cups and bake for approx. 15-20 min.

Yogurts

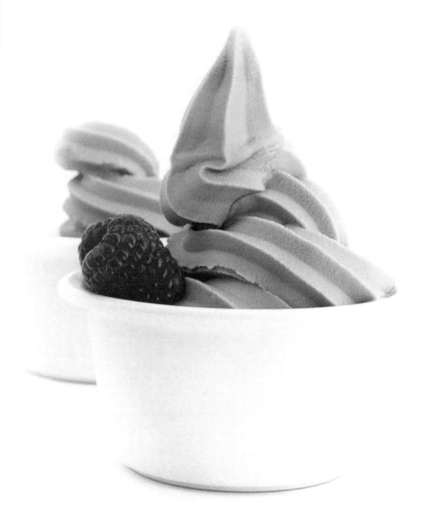

Health benefits of Greek yogurt and kefir: You can count yogurt as a calcium rich bone builder. It provides the same amount of calcium as an 8 oz glass of milk. Greek yogurt with live cultures contain "good" bacteria, the kind that offer numerous health benefits, including boosting the immune system, alleviating diarrhea caused by some infections or treatment with antibiotics, relieving constipation, and even reducing the risk of developing colon cancer. As far as yogurt's immune benefits go, more than 79 percent of the body's natural immune defenses are located in the digestive tract. Building up the "good" bacteria that come from live Greek yogurt and kefir will help boost production of important immune system compounds.

7.5 Yogurts

Yogurt is another fast and simple way to get protein, and you can add your own flare by adding your choice of fruits and nuts.

7.5.1 SIMPLE / QUICK ON THE GO GREEK YOGURT

Nutritional Information: *(3 oz. protein, 1 tbsp. fat, ¼ cup fruit)*

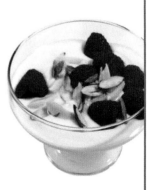

- ✓ ½ cup plain Greek yogurt
- ✓ Handful of chopped nuts of choice
- ✓ ¼ cup fruit of choice (berries and bananas are my favorite)

✓ 1 tsp. Stevia, maple syrup or honey

7.5.2 YOGURT DREAM

Nutritional Information: *(3 oz. protein, 1 tbsp. fat, ¼ cup fruit)*

- ✓ ½ cup plain Greek yogurt
- ✓ 1/8 cup chopped raw nuts (pumpkin, sesame, almonds, pecans, walnuts) pick two different kinds
- ✓ ¼ cup berries (banana or both)
- ✓ 1 tsp. maple syrup

Mix and enjoy in place of ice cream. To add carb & fruit choose: oatmeal with fruit or Ezekiel toast with a side of fruit or topped with fruit.

7.5.3 SIMPLE ORANGE YOGURT

Nutritional Information: *(4 oz. protein, ½ cup fruit)*

- ✓ 3 oz. Greek yogurt
- ✓ ½ cup orange segments (place on top)
- ✓ 1 tsp. honey

7.5.4 EZEKIEL BREAD TOAST WITH GREEK YOGURT

Nutritional Information: *(3 oz. protein, ¼ cup fruit, ½ cup carbs)*

- ✓ Toast 1 slice. Ezekiel bread

- ✓ add 1 tsp. of honey (if you want to add your fat, you could add 1 tbsp. peanut butter)
- ✓ ½ cup Greek yogurt
- ✓ topped with ¼ cup fruit of choice & 1 tsp. of Stevia

Smoothies and Power Drinks

7.6 Smoothies & Power Drinks

Smoothies and shakes are another way to ensure protein and veggies to start your day.

Spinach masks well in smoothies/shakes and so add a 1/2 of spinach or kale, to your choice of whey protein powder, ¼ cup of fruit of choice, ice, water, or if you need extra calories and fat add ¼ cup almond /coconut / rice milk or raw peanut butter

NOTE: In most of my smoothies I add **Amazing Grass** superfood blend. Chocolate flavored in my chocolate ones and berry flavor in my berry or fruit blends.

Most green drinks make 2 servings. I either share or save the rest to drink later in the day as a snack. I mix this in my **Blendtec** blender. You can also use your juicer or high powered blender for all green drinks listed. I personally start my day with a green drink. It has done wonders for my skin and my energy!

7.6.1 CHOCOLATE DELIGHT SMOOTHIE

Nutritional Information: *(3 oz. protein, ½ cup veggies, ¼ cup fruit)*

- ✓ ½ cup spinach or kale leaves
- ✓ 1 tbsp. cocoa powder
- ✓ 1 scoop of chocolate whey protein
- ✓ ½ large or 1 small banana (you can substitute banana for ¼ cup frozen/reg. cherries or blueberries)
- ✓ Handful of ice and 1 cup water

Blend and enjoy!

> Chia seeds, ground flax seeds, spinach and kale are great health boosters you can add to any smoothie for a health kick.

7.6.2 BANANA SMOOTHIE

Nutritional Information: 1 smoothie = *(½ cup fruit, 3 oz. protein) Makes 2 smoothies*

- ✓ 1 medium banana
- ✓ ½ cup almond/rice/coconut milk
- ✓ ½ cup water
- ✓ ¼ cup strawberries
- ✓ 1-2 scoop whey protein
- ✓ Ice (if desired)

Blend and enjoy!

7.6.3 NECTARINE SMOOTHIE

Nutritional Information: *(¼ cup fruit, 3 oz. protein)*

- ✓ 1 chilled nectarine
- ✓ 1 scoop of vanilla whey protein
- ✓ Handful of ice
- ✓ 1 cup water

Blend and serve!

7.6.4 ANTI-AGING SMOOTHIE

Nutritional Information: *(½ cup veggies, 3 oz. protein, ½ tbsp. fat, ¼ cup fruit)*

- ✓ 1/3 cup unsweetened almond milk
- ✓ 2/3 cup water
- ✓ ½ cup of kale
- ✓ 1 scoop chocolate protein powder
- ✓ ¼ cup frozen cherries or blueberries
  6 ice cubes

Blend and enjoy, under 100 calories and yummy too!

7.6.5 ORANGE JULIUS

Nutritional Information: 1 smoothie *(½ cup fruit, 1 oz. protein, ½ tbsp. fat)*

Makes 4 servings

This smoothie is good for you and your skin!

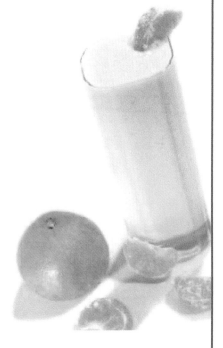

- ✓ Take 1 fresh orange peeled and segmented, but in blender
- ✓ Add ¼ cup 100% orange concentrate
- ✓ 1 tsp. of vanilla
- ✓ 2 scoops of vanilla whey protein

✓ 3 tsp. Stevia or 3 Stevia packets
✓ ½ cup water 1 cup coconut or almond milk
✓ Handful of ice

Blend and serve. Yum!

7.6.6 WATERMELON BANANA BOOSTER

Nutritional Information: *(3 oz. protein, ½ cup fruit, 1 tbsp. fat if you use milk)*

✓ ¼ cup seedless watermelon
✓ ¼ cup banana
✓ 1 cup plain almond milk or half milk/half water or all water
✓ 1 scoop whey protein/ice cubes

Blend and enjoy!

7.6.7 GREEN PROTEIN POWER

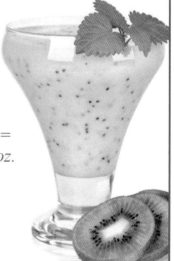

Nutritional Information: 1 drink = *(1/4 cup fruit, ¼ cup veggies, 2 oz. protein)*

Makes 2 drinks

✓ 2 kiwi fruit
✓ 1 med. banana
✓ 1/2cup spinach
✓ 1 scoop vanilla whey protein
✓ add 1 tbsp. flaxseed-optional
✓ 1 cup water

✓ Ice cubes

7.6.8 CRANBERRY FAT FLUSH DRINK

Nutritional Information: *(flavors your water & is good for you)*

- ✓ ½ cup unsweetened cranberry juice
- ✓ 1 tbsp. grounds flaxseed
- ✓ Mixed with 1 liter of water

Drink 1 daily.

7.6.9 GREEN JUICE JOLT

Nutritional Information: 1 drink = *(½ cup veggies, ¼ cup fruit)* Super good and super good for you!

Makes 2 drinks

- ✓ ¼ cup spinach
- ✓ 1 med. carrot
- ✓ 1 apple
- ✓ ½ large lemon squeezed
- ✓ 1/2 pc. ginger peeled'
- ✓ Handful of Ice

Blend together and enjoy!

7.6.10 BERRY MILK SHAKE

Nutritional Information: *(3 oz. protein, ½ tbsp. fat if you add the milk, ¼ cup fruit)*

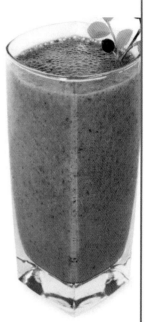

- ✓ ½ cup almond /rice /coconut milk
- ✓ ½ cup water
- ✓ 1 scoop whey protein powder
- ✓ 2 strawberries
- ✓ ¼ cup blueberries

Blend and enjoy!

NOTE: You can use water instead of almond/rice/or coconut milk if you do not want the extra calories.

7.6.11 CHOCOLATE AVOCADO DREAM

Nutritional Information: 1 drink = *(1 tbsp. fat, ¼ cup fruit)*

Makes 2 drinks

- ✓ 1 cup milk/almond /coconut milk
- ✓ 2 tbsp. cocoa powder
- ✓ 1 ripe banana
- ✓ 1 avocado
- ✓ 1 cup ice

Blend all together for an amazing smooth chocolate shake and enjoy!

7.6.12 POWERED UP CHOCOLATE AVOCADO DREAM

Nutritional Information: 1 drink = *(1 tbsp. fat, ¼ cup fruit, ½ cup veggies)*

Makes 2 drinks

- ✓ 1 cup milk/almond /coconut milk
- ✓ 2 tbsp. cocoa powder
- ✓ 1-2 scoop chocolate whey protein
- ✓ ¼ cup cucumber
- ✓ ½ cup spinach
- ✓ 1 ripe banana
- ✓ 1 avocado
- ✓ 3 figs (optional)
- ✓ 1 cup ice

Blend all together. Enjoy! It will sometimes come out like chocolate pudding. YUM!

7.6.13 GREEN MAGIC

Nutritional Information: 1 drink = *(2 oz protein, ½ - ¾ cup veggies, ¼ cup fruit)*

Makes 2 drinks

- ✓ 1 cup water
- ✓ Handful kale
- ✓ Handful spinach
- ✓ Thumb tip size of fresh ginger
- ✓ ¼ cup cucumber
- ✓ 1 tbsp. hemp or chia seeds or both

✓ ½ pear or apple

Blend together and enjoy!

7.6.14 MORNING SUPERCHARGE

Nutritional Information: 1 drink = *(1cup of amazing veggies)*

  - ✓ 1 cup water
  - ✓ Handful kale and spinach (use both or 1 of them depending on what you have in the fridge)
  - ✓ ¼ cup fresh parsley
  - ✓ ¼ cup fresh cilantro
  - ✓ ½ cup cucumber
  - ✓ Pinch cayenne pepper
  - ✓ Squeeze ½ lemon

Blend and enjoy this Superfood, Supercharge Drink that will chase any zit away!

7.6.15 RASPBERRY BASIL SMOOTHIE

Nutritional Information: 1 drink = *(½ cup fruit)*

Makes 2 drinks

  - ✓ 2 ½ cups frozen/fresh raspberries
  - ✓ 1 cup almond milk or water
  - ✓ 1 red apple
  - ✓ 3 tbsp. packed fresh basil
  - ✓ Zest of 1 lemon
  - ✓ 1 tsp. honey (optional)

Without peeling the apple, coarsely chop it and add to the blender. Add the rest of the ingredients and blend until smooth. Serve quickly with a sprig of basil and a couple of fresh raspberries as garnish.

7.6.16 BERRY-PROTEIN SMOOTHIE

Nutritional Information: 1 drink = *(3 oz protein, ¼ cup veggies, ½ cup fruit)*

Makes 2 drinks

- ✓ ¼ cup hemp seeds
- ✓ 1 scoop vanilla whey protein
- ✓ ½ cup frozen mixed berries
- ✓ 1 ripe banana
- ✓ ½ cup spinach or kale
- ✓ ½ cup water

Combine all ingredients in a blender, and blend until smooth.

7.6.17 MANGO-COCONUT WATER SMOOTHIE

These nutritious combos of fruit, veggies, proteins, and healthy fats make delicious snacks or quick lunches on the go.

Nutritional Information: 1 drink = *(½ cup fruit, ¼ cup veggies)*

Makes 2 drinks

- ✓ 1 cup ripe mango chunks (from 1-2 mangos)
- ✓ 2-3 tbsp. fresh lime juice

- ✓ ½ cup spinach
- ✓ 1 cup unsweetened coconut water
- ✓ Pinch of cayenne powder

Combine all ingredients in a blender, and blend until smooth.

NOTE: To add 3 oz protein, you can add whey protein powder or 1-2 tbsp. hemp or chia seeds to the recipe.

7.6.18 GREEN SMOOTHIE

Nutritional Information: 1 drink = *(1 cup veggies, ½ cup fruit)*

Makes 2 drinks

- ✓ 1 cup kale or collard greens firmly packed, stems removed, coarsely chopped (4 oz)
- ✓ 1 Granny Smith apple, coarsely chopped
- ✓ 1 ripe banana
- ✓ ½ cup loosely packed fresh flat-leaf parsley leaves
- ✓ 2 ¼ cups water

Combine all ingredients in a blender, and blend until smooth. If the mixture is too thick, add a little more water.

NOTE: To add 3 oz protein, you can add whey protein powder or 1-2 tbsp. hemp or chia seeds to the recipe.

7.6.19 BLUEBERRY-ALMOND BUTTER SMOOTHIE

Nutritional Information: 1 drink = *(1 tbsp. fat, ¼ cup veggies, ½ cup fruit, 3 oz protein)*

Makes 2 drinks

- ✓ ½ cup frozen blueberries
- ✓ 2 tbsp. almond butter
- ✓ 1 ripe banana
- ✓ ½ cup spinach
- ✓ 1 tbsp. lemon juice
- ✓ 2 tbsp. flaxseeds or chia seeds
- ✓ 3 dates (Medjool or Deglet), pitted
- ✓ 2 cups water

Combine all ingredients in a blender, and blend until smooth.

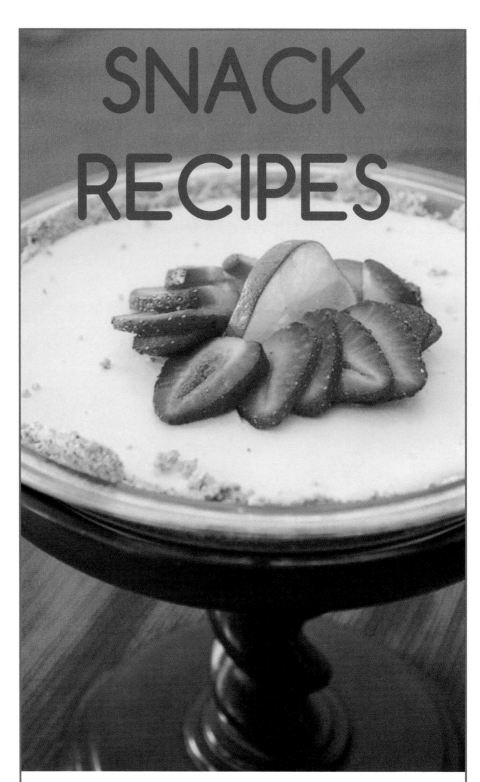

SNACK RECIPES

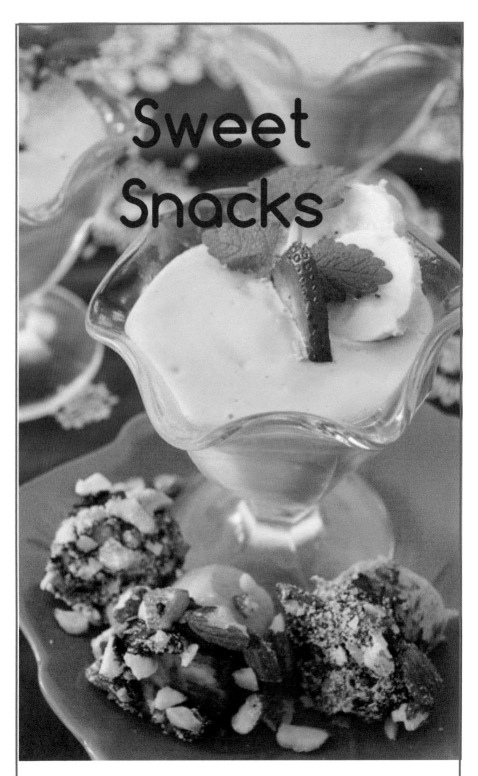

Sweet
Snacks

7.7 Sweet Easy Treats

7.7.1 TROPICAL TRAIL MIX

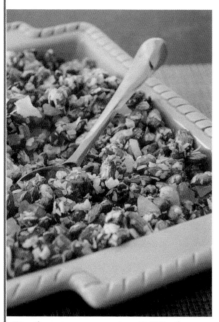

Nutritional Information: *(½ cup = approximately 2 oz. protein, ¼ cup fruit, 1 tbsp. fat)*

- ✓ 2 cups raw almonds
- ✓ 1 cup raw cashews
- ✓ 1 cup unsweetened coconut flakes
- ✓ 1 cup dried pineapple and papaya
- ✓ ¼ cup honey
- ✓ ½ tsp. allspice and ginger

Preheat oven to 350-degrees. Line the baking sheet with parchment paper. In small saucepan heat honey and spices together over low heat. In a large bowl, combine almonds, cashews and then add mixture and toss together.

Spread on baking sheet and bake for 15-20 minutes. Cook and let cool 3 minutes, and then toss with coconut, and fruit, store in airtight container after cooled completely.

7.7.2 PLUM BRUSCHETTA

Nutritional Information: *(½ cup carbs, ¼ cup fruit, 1-2 oz. protein)*

- ✓ 2 tbsp. ricotta cheese
- ✓ 1 slc. toasted Ezekiel bread
- ✓ 1 plum
- ✓ 1/2 tsp. honey
- ✓ pinch nutmeg

Mix 2 tbsp. non-fat ricotta cheese with a pinch of nutmeg, spread over toasted Ezekiel bread. Top with a sliced plum and drizzle ½ tsp. honey on top.

7.7.3 APPLE WITH ALMOND BUTTER

Nutritional Information: *(½ cup fruit, 1 tbsp. fat)*

- ✓ ½ apple sliced
- ✓ Add 2 tsp. almond butter or peanut butter

7.7.4 COCONUT COVERED TREAT

Nutritional Information: *(1/2 cup fruit)*

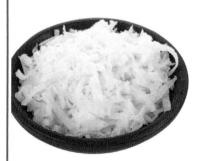

- ✓ ½ cup pineapple or mixed melon
- ✓ Topped with 2 tsp. shredded coconut

7.7.5 CINNAMON STRIPS

Nutritional Information: *(½ cup carbs, 2 oz. protein)*

- ✓ 1 Small gluten free tortilla, cut into wedges
- ✓ Sprinkle with cinnamon
- ✓ 1/3 cup plain Greek yogurt
- ✓ 1 tsp. honey

Bake at 350-degrees for 10 minutes. Dip cooled chips in 1/3 cup Greek yogurt with 1 tsp. honey

7.7.6 WARM APPLE

Nutritional Information: *(½ cup fruit)*

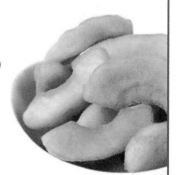

- ✓ 1 apple (sliced)
- ✓ cinnamon
- ✓ 1 tsp. Stevia

Boil for 1 minute, drain and sprinkle with cinnamon and stevia.

7.7.7 CHOCOLATE BANANA

Nutritional Information: *1/2 banana (¼ cup fruit, ½ tbs. fat)*

- ✓ ½ banana
- ✓ 1 tsp. almond butter
- ✓ 2 tsp. unsweetened shredded coconut
- ✓ unsweetened cocoa powder

Slice banana in half, spread almond butter on both sides and sprinkle with coconut. Freeze 1-3 hours. Dust with a pinch of unsweetened cocoa powder. This is one of my kid's favorites and mine!

7.7.8 CHOCOLATE APPLE PROTEIN BARS

Nutritional Information: *1 nutrition bar (3 oz. protein, ¼ cup carbs, 1 tbs. fat, minimal fruit)*

- ✓ 2 cups rolled oats
- ✓ ½ cup natural nut butter
- ✓ 4 tbsp. chia seeds
- ✓ 4 scoops chocolate protein powder
- ✓ ½ cup unsweetened applesauce

Combine all ingredients together. Place in an 8'' sq. baking dish with parchment paper. Put in the freezer for 30 min. Remove and cut into 6 bars.

7.7.9 CHOCOLATE COVERED ALMONDS

Nutritional Information: *5 almonds (1 tbsp. fat, 2 oz protein)*

- ✓ 10 raw unsalted almonds
- ✓ 4 squares of dark chocolate (65%+)

Heat up the dark chocolate until soft, put almonds in and mix around until the almonds are coated with chocolate. Place on parchment paper until dried. Yummy, quick treat.

7.7.10 FRESH FRUIT WITH APPLESAUCE SWEENTENED TAHINI

Nutritional Information: *(¾ cup fruit, 3 oz protein)*

Makes 3 servings- you can share or save to eat later or another day

- ✓ ¼ cup tahini
- ✓ ½ cup unsweetened applesauce
- ✓ 1 tbsp. honey
- ✓ 2 tbsp. water
- ✓ 3 cups sliced fruit, such as mango, grapes, plums, berries, and citrus
- ✓ ¼ cup unsweetened coconut flakes

Combine tahini, applesauce, honey, and water in a food processor. Pulse until smooth. Arrange fruit in serving bowls. Drizzle tahini sauce and top with toasted coconut.

7.7.11 CARIBBEAN DREAM

Nutritional Information: *(½ cup = ½ cup fruit)*

Makes 4-8 servings- great side dish to take to a party!

- ✓ 2 apples, chopped finely
- ✓ 1 kiwi, sliced thinly
- ✓ 1 cup watermelon, chopped fine
- ✓ 1 mango, chopped
- ✓ 1 peach, chopped
- ✓ ½ cup lemon juice
- ✓ ¼ cup coconut milk

Mix all the fruit together and dress with the lemon juice and coconut milk. Toss gently.

NOTE: I would also add berries and/or bananas, plums instead of watermelon and peaches if you like.

7.7.12 CHOCOLATE CHIP COOKIE DOUGH

Nutritional Information: *(3 oz protein, 1 tbsp. fat- dependent on if you use almond butter and almonds)*

- ✓ ½ cup Greek yogurt
- ✓ 1 tsp. – 1 tbsp. almond butter (optional)
- ✓ 1 tsp. stevia
- ✓ 1 tsp. slivered almonds (optional)
- ✓ 1 tsp. vanilla
- ✓ 1 tbsp. dark chocolate chips (try to get 70% or higher cocoa chips)

Mix all together. Quick and easy and satisfies the need for a sweet treat like cookie dough.

7.8 Smoothies / Power Drinks / Warm Drinks

Smoothies and shakes are another way to ensure protein and veggies to start your day.

Spinach masks well in smoothies/shakes and so add a 1/2 of spinach or kale, to your choice of whey protein powder, ¼ cup of fruit of choice, ice, water, or if you need extra calories and fat add ¼ cup almond /coconut / rice milk.

7.8.1 CHOCOLATE DELIGHT SMOOTHIE

Nutritional Information: *(3 oz. protein, ½ cup veggies, ¼ cup fruit)*

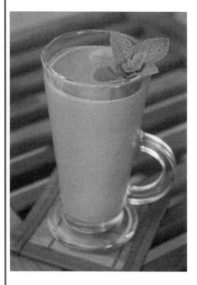

✓   ½ cup spinach or kale leaves
✓   1 tbsp. cocoa powder
✓   1 scoop of chocolate whey protein
✓   ½ large or 1 small banana (you can substitute banana for ¼ cup frozen/reg. cherries or blueberries)
✓   Handful of ice
✓   1 cup of water

Blend and enjoy!

7.8.2 BANANA SMOOTHIE

Nutritional Information: 1 smoothie = *(½ cup fruit, 3 oz. protein)*

Makes up to 2 smoothies

✓ 1 medium banana
✓ ½ cup almond/rice/coconut milk
✓ ¼ cup strawberries
✓ 1-2 scoop whey protein
    ½ cup water
    Ice (if desired)
Blend.

7.8.3 ORANGE JULIUS

Nutritional Information: *(½ cup fruit, 1 oz. protein, ½ tbsp. fat)*

Makes 4 servings

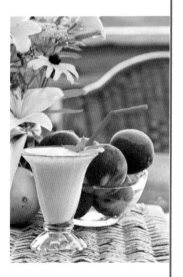

- ✓ Take 1 fresh orange peeled and segmented, but in blender.
- ✓ Add ¼ cup 100% orange concentrate
- ✓ 1 tsp. of vanilla
- ✓ 1 scoop of vanilla whey protein
- ✓ 3 tsp. Stevia or 3 Stevia packets
  ½ cup water 1 cup coconut or almond milk
  Handful of ice

This smoothie is good for you and your skin! Blend and serve. Yum!

7.8.4 NECTARINE SMOOTHIE

Nutritional Information: *(¼ cup fruit, 3 oz. protein)*

- ✓ 1 chilled nectarine
- ✓ 1 scoop of vanilla whey protein
- ✓ Handful of ice
- ✓ 1 cup water

Blend and serve.

7.8.5 ANTI-AGING SMOOTHIE

Nutritional Information: *(½ cup veggies, 3 oz. protein, ½ tbsp. fat, ¼ cup fruit)*

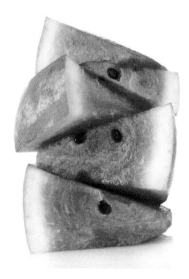

- ✓ 1/3 cup unsweetened almond milk
  - ✓ ½ cup of kale
    - ✓ 1 scoop chocolate protein powder
      - ✓ ¼ cup frozen cherries or blueberries
      2/3 cup water
      6 ice cubes

      Blend and enjoy, under 100 calories and yummy too!

7.8.6 WATERMELON BANANA BOOSTER

Nutritional Information: *(3 oz. protein, ½ cup fruit, 1 tbsp. fat if you use milk)*

- ✓ ¼ cup seedless watermelon
- ✓ ¼ cup banana
- ✓ 1 cup plain almond milk or half milk/half water or all water
- ✓ 1 scoop whey protein/ice cubes

Blend and enjoy!

7.8.7 GREEN PROTEIN POWER

Nutritional Information: 1 drink = *(¼ cup fruit, ¼ cup veggies, 2 oz. protein)*

Makes 2 drinks

- ✓ 2 kiwi fruit
- ✓ 1 med. banana
- ✓ 1 cup spinach
- ✓ 1 scoop vanilla whey protein (add tbsp. flaxseed-optional)
- ✓ 1 cup water
- ✓ Ice cubes

7.8.8 GREEN JUICE JOLT

Nutritional Information: 1 drink = *(½ cup veggies, ¼ cup fruit)*

Makes 2 drinks

Super good and super good for you! Mix in blender.

- ✓ ¼ cup spinach
- ✓ 1 med. carrot
- ✓ 1 apple
- ✓ ½ large lemon squeezed
- ✓ 1/2 pc. ginger peeled
- ✓ Ice

7.8.9 CRANBERRY FAT FLUSH DRINK

Nutritional Information: *(flavors your water & is good for you)*

- ✓ ½ cup unsweetened cranberry juice
- ✓ 1 tbsp. ground flaxseed

Mixed with 1 liter of water and have 1 daily!

7.8.10 BERRY MILK SHAKE

Nutritional Information: *(3 oz. protein, ½ Tbsp. fat if you add the milk, ¼ cup fruit)*

- ✓ ½ cup almond/rice/coconut milk
- ✓ 1 scoop whey protein powder
- ✓ 2 strawberries
- ✓ ¼ cup blueberries
- ✓ ½ cup water

Blend and enjoy!

NOTE: You can use water in place of almond / rice/ or coconut milk if you do not want the extra calories.

7.8.11 HOT CHOCOLATE

Nutritional Information: *(1 tsp. fat) (if Superfood blend is added, then add ¼ cup veggies)*

- ✓ Take 1 cup of almond/coconut milk
- ✓ Add 2 tbsp. unsweetened cocoa powder

✓ Mix and heat up on stove until hot
✓ Add 2 tsp. honey (optional)

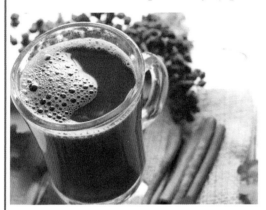

NOTE: I add 1 scoop of chocolate - amazing grass Superfood blend to this drink for extra nutritional value. My kids love it too!

7.9 Cookie / Bars / Power Bites

7.9.1 CHOCOLATE PEANUT BUTTER BITES

Nutritional Information: *2 ball = (3 oz. protein, 1 tbsp. fat, ¼ cup carbs)*

Makes approximately 25 balls

- ✓ 1 cup natural peanut butter or almond butter
- ✓ ¼ cup honey
- ✓ 3 cups slow cooked oatmeal (you can ground this up in blender if you want a cookie dough texture and then add)
- ✓ 2-3 scoops vanilla or chocolate whey protein (I love chocolate)
  1/3 cup water

Mix, roll into 1 inch balls, eat or freeze. Enjoy!

Optional: You can roll in coconut or add dark cocoa nibs (65% higher chocolate chips or cocoa nibs) to the mixture.

NOTE: I love to freeze these and take them out as a frozen treat. I have children and so these are in my home at least half of the month. I do not make cookies, this is what my kids think are cookies! In all of our opinion's these taste just as good and feel even better after you eat them!

7.9.2 COOKIE DOUGH

Nutritional Information: 1 ball (*1 tbsp. fat, 1/8 cup carbs*)

- ✓ Pulse or puree 2/3 cup almonds
- ✓ 2/3 cup walnuts
- ✓ 2/3 cup oats
- ✓ Add to mixture ¼ cup honey or agave
- ✓ 1 tsp. cinnamon
- ✓ 1 tsp. vanilla
- ✓ Handful of dark chocolate nibs

Mix all above ingredients. Make into 1-inch balls, place in the freezer, and enjoy!

7.9.3 FRUIT & NUT ENERGY BARS

Nutritional Information: 2 balls= (*2 oz. protein, ¼ cup fruit, 1 tsp. fat*)
Makes approx. 5 bars or 10 balls

- ✓ 8 prunes/plumes
- ✓ 5 figs (optional)
- ✓ ¼ cup of almonds
- ✓ 1 cup slow cooked oats blended into powder
- ✓ 1 scoop of chocolate whey protein

Blend/pulse in blender prunes/plumes, figs and almonds. Then add oats and whey protein.

NOTE: Very sticky consistency and the nuts are not evenly chopped, roll into balls or bars, wrap individual bars in plastic wrap, and then place in freezer until ready to eat.

7.9.4 RICH COCOA BITES

Nutritional Information: *(1 ball = 2 oz. protein, ½ tbsp. fat, ¼ cup fruit).*

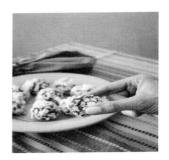

- ✓ ¼ c dates
- ✓ ½ cup oats
- ✓ ¼ cup raisins
- ✓ ¼ cup mixed nuts (raw and unsalted)
- ✓ 2 heaped organic cocoa powder
- ✓ 1 tsp. cinnamon

Mix all ingredients in a blender.

Optional: Add 100% pure raw cacao nibs or for protein 1 scoop of whey protein. Add (while blending) some water for a sticky consistency.

Take out small heaps with a tablespoon and roll balls with your hands. Roll in shredded coconut (preferably raw unsweetened).

Store in the fridge for at least one hour, in an open container, so that excessive moisture can escape. I love to freeze these and eat as a cold yummy treat. Great after dinner snack.

7.9.5 PEANUT BUTTER CUP BITES

Nutritional Information: *(2 balls = 3 oz. protein, 1 tbsp. fat, ¼ cup carbs)*

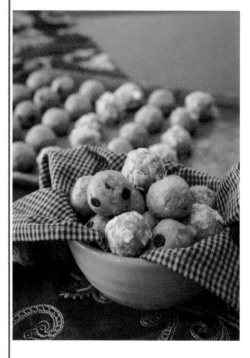

- ✓ ¾ cup raw peanut butter
- ✓ ¼ cup honey
- ✓ ¼ cup coarsely chopped assorted raw nuts (I use sunflower seeds, & chopped almonds)
- ✓ 2 -3 cup oats
- ✓ 1 scoop chocolate whey protein
- ✓ 1/3 cup water if needed to moisten enough to make a ball with hands.

Mix together, roll into cookie balls and place in the freezer. Eat when you want.

7.9.6 HEALTHY PUMPKIN PROTEIN COOKIES

Nutritional Information: *(1 cookie = ½ cup carb, 2 oz. protein, ¼ cup fruit, 1 tbsp. fat).* You can eat these for breakfast!

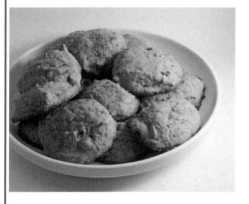

- ✓ 1 ½ cup slow cooked oats
- ✓ 1 cup almond or raw peanut butter
- ✓ ¼ cup honey
- ✓ ½ cup pumpkin
- ✓ ½ cup unsweetened apple sauce
- ✓ 1 cup protein powder (preferably vanilla)
- ✓ 1 tbsp. pumpkin spice
- ✓ 1 tbsp. cinnamon

Mix and bake at 350-degrees for 20 minutes. You can make these into bars & cut them and freeze remaining bars or make individual round cookie shapes.

NOTE: This contains 6 ingredients, but too good to leave out!

7.9.7 NO BAKE APPLE CHOCOLATE BARS

Nutritional Information: (*1 bar = ¼ cup carbs, 1 tbsp. fat, 3 oz. protein, 1/8 cup fruit)* (very minimal)

- ✓ 2 cups rolled oats
- ✓ ½ cup natural nut butter

- ✓ ¼ cup coconut or grape seed oil
- ✓ 4 scoops chocolate protein powder
- ✓ ½ cup unsweetened applesauce

Line an 8" pan with parchment paper, combine all ingredients, pour ingredients into pan, freeze for 30 minutes, then remove and cut into 6 bars.

7.10 Yogurt / Cottage Cheese

7.10.1 SPICED KEFIR

Nutritional Information: *(3 oz. protein, ½ tsp. fat)*

- ✓ 3 oz. low fat kefir sprinkled with
- ✓ 1/8 tsp. cinnamon or cardamom
- ✓ 1 tsp. flaxseed meal or chia seeds

7.10.2 KEY LIME PIE

Nutritional Information: *(3 oz. protein)*

- ✓ ½ cup plain Greek yogurt
- ✓ Squeeze ½ of a fresh lime into yogurt
- ✓ 1 tsp. Stevia

Mix and enjoy!

7.10.3 CHIA PUDDING

Nutritional Information: ½ cup prepared = *(3-4 oz. protein, 1 tbsp. fat)*

- ✓ 3/4 cup Chia seeds
- ✓ 2 cups almond milk
- ✓ 1 tsp. maple syrup
- ✓ 1 tsp. vanilla extract to taste
- ✓ dash of cinnamon

Chia Seeds Fun Facts: These little seeds are bursting with so many health benefits. They help you lose weight, balance blood sugar, add healthy omega 3's, and have age defying antioxidants.

Mix the ingredients together in a Mason jar and let chill in fridge for 30 minutes. The Chia seeds will swell and absorb the milk turning it to a pudding.

I add 100% raw cocoa, but I love the chocolate taste and it has antioxidants to boot.

7.10.4 CHOCOLATE POWER PUDDING

Nutritional Information: 1 serving = *(3 oz. protein, 1/8 cup fruit) (very minimal)*
Makes 2 servings

- ✓ 2 scoop chocolate protein powder
- ✓ 1 cup plain Greek yogurt
- ✓ 2 tsp. unsweetened cocoa powder
- ✓ 1 packet of Stevia (1 tsp.)
- ✓ 6 raspberries

Mix and eat.

NOTE: For extra energy and nutrient value, you can add Chia seeds.

7.10.5 ON THE GO COTTAGE CHEESE

Nutritional Information: *(3 oz. protein, with ¼ cup fruit)*

- ✓ 3 oz. cottage cheese
- ✓ ¼ cup apples slices

7.11 Ice Cream Recipes

7.11.1 PEPPERMINT PROTEIN ICE CREAM

Nutritional Information: *(½ cup = 2 oz. protein, ½ tbsp. fat)*

- ✓ 1 cup unsweetened vanilla or original almond milk
- ✓ 1 scoop vanilla whey protein powder
- ✓ ¼ tsp. peppermint extract (or any flavoring extract you prefer)
- ✓ ¼ cup unsweetened Greek yogurt

Mix everything together in a blender; pour in sandwich-sized bag. Fill a gallon size bag half way with ice. Add ½ cup table salt. Place the small bag into the large bag and seal. Shake the bag vigorously for 5 minutes.

This is super fun for family and kids. Remove bag, rinse salt off bag and serve. You can serve with crushed peppermint candy.

7.11.2 PEANUT BUTTER ICE CREAM

Nutritional Information: *(1 tbsp. fat, 3 oz. protein, ¼ cup fruit)*

- ✓ ½ banana
- ✓ 2 tbsp. of crunchy (or nutty) peanut butter
- ✓ ½ tsp. of vanilla extract
- ✓ 1 scoop of the pure protein powder

Freeze the banana. I suggest you break the banana into smaller pieces, then place it into a plastic container and keep it in the freezer overnight. Place frozen banana into blender, add peanut butter, ½ tsp. vanilla, and 1 scoop of pure protein powder. Place in your favorite bowl and add cinnamon on top if you like. Yum!

7.11.3 BANANA NICE CREAM

Nutritional Information: *(1 tbsp. fat, ½ cup fruit)*

Makes 2 drinks

- ✓ 2 frozen bananas
- ✓ 1 cup unsweetened vanilla almond milk
- ✓ 2 tbsp. almond butter

Blend. Enjoy!

7.11.4 SPINACH ICE CREAM

You and your toughest critique will love this!
NOTE: You will need a **Blentec** blender or Vitamix to make this recipe

Nutritional Information: *(3 oz protein, ½ cup veggies, ¼ cup fruit)*

Makes 4 servings

- ✓ ¾ cup almond or coconut milk
- ✓ ¼ cup honey
- ✓ ½ banana
- ✓ ½ cup vanilla whey protein
- ✓ 2 cups spinach, lightly packed
- ✓ 1 ½ tbsp. vanilla extract
- ✓ 2 ½ cup ice cubes

Enjoy!

7.12 Pies / Brownies / Cobbler

7.12.1 AMAZING APPLE CRISP

Nutritional Information: *(½ cup = ½ cup fruit, 1/8 cup carbs) if you add yogurt, then add 2 oz. protein)*

- ✓ 3 apples (diced)
- ✓ 1 tbsp. cinnamon
- ✓ 1 tbsp. apple cider vinegar (this has some great health proponents)
- ✓ ½ cup oats
- ✓ 1 tbsp. stevia
- ✓ 1 tbsp. water

Mix and bake on 350-degrees for 30 minutes. You can serve this with a 1/2 cup of Greek yogurt.

7.12.2   SIMPLE CHOCOLATE

Nutritional Information: (*1 tbsp. fat*)
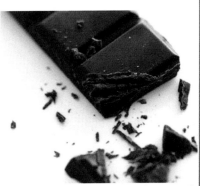
- ✓ 1 square of 70% or higher dark chocolate

Only eat this if really craving something simple and something chocolate.

7.12.3 WARM, MOIST CHOCOLATIE BROWNIES

Nutritional Information: (*1 sq. inch = ¼ cup carbs, ¼ cup fruit, 3 oz. protein*)

- ✓ 1 cup oat flour (or 1/2 cup oat flour & 1/2 cup almond flour)
- ✓ 3 tbsp. unsweetened cocoa powder (100% cacao)
- ✓ 2 scoops chocolate protein powder
- ✓ 1/8 cup Stevia (or 1/4 cup Splenda)
- ✓ 8 oz. berry flavored applesauce (or baby food)
- ✓ 4 egg whites or 2 whole eggs

Preheat oven to 350-degrees. Mix dry ingredients (oat flour, chocolate whey powder, baking cocoa together in a large bowl. Mix wet ingredients (egg whites, berry applesauce, Stevia) together in a medium-sized bowl. Add wet ingredients to the dry ingredients. Oil a 9x9 pan with coconut oil or non-stick spray and spread mixture evenly among pan.

Bake for 20-25 minutes. For an extra delicious treat, try topping with a small serving of peanut, or almond butter, or coconut flakes. Even as is, these bad boys will rock your socks.

7.12.4 WARM FALL APPLE COBBLER

Nutritional Information: *(½ cup of this mixture = 1 tbsp. fat, ½ cup fruit, 1/8 cup carbs)*

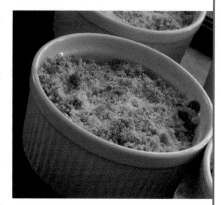

- ✓ Boil 1 lb. chopped apples
- ✓ 1 cup pear or berries or whatever fruit you prefer
- ✓ ¼ cup oatmeal
- ✓ ¼ cup quinoa flour
- ✓ ¼ cup chopped dates
- ✓ 1/8 cup chopped almonds

Mix together like a crumble with 3 tbsp. olive oil or grape-seed oil. Place cooked fruit in sprayed pan, sprinkle 2 tsp. cinnamon on top and then sprinkle crumble mixture on top! Cook at 350-degrees for 25 minutes.

NOTE: To add protein, you can top with Greek yogurt & honey.

7.12.5 KEY LIME CHEESECAKE

Nutritional Information: *(1 serving = (3 oz. protein, 1 tbsp. fat),* if you top with ¼ cup fresh fruit then add ¼ cup fruit.

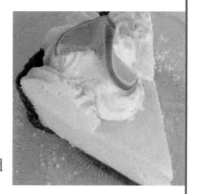

Crust:

- ✓ 1½ cup finely chopped walnuts
- ✓ 2 tbsp. coconut oil
- ✓ 2 tbsp. honey

Press all the above ingredients together and press in the bottom of your pie pan.

NOTE: It will seem not fully compact, but once you add pie filling, it all comes out nicely after cooked.

Filling:

- ✓ 1 cup cottage cheese (blended until smooth)
- ✓ 1 cup plain Greek yogurt
- ✓ 2 limes juiced
- ✓ ½ cup Stevia or ¼ cup honey
- ✓ 2 eggs or 1 whole egg and 2 egg whites

Mix all ingredients together until smooth. Pour into crust. Place in 350-degrees oven for 20-30 minutes or until set. Let cool and refrigerate a few hours before serving. Garnish with sliced strawberries and drizzle with honey or melted dark chocolate (optional).

Savory Dips
& Snacks

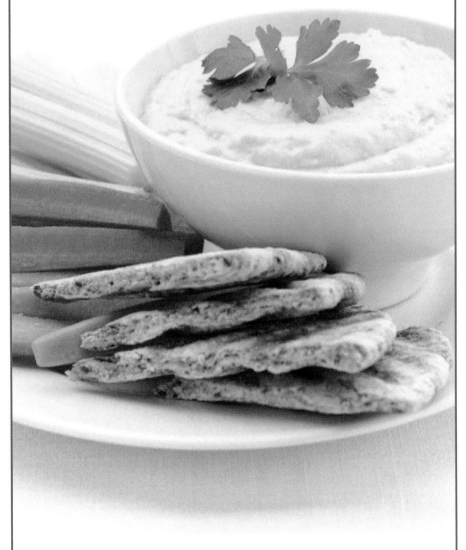

7.13 Savory Dips & Snacks

7.13.1 AVOCADO HUMMUS

Nutritional Information: *(1/2 cup veggies, 1 tbsp. fat, 1/8 cup carbs)*

- ✓ ¼ cup avocado (puree)
- ✓ 2 tbsp. hummus
- ✓ ½ tsp. lemon juice
- ✓ 1/2 cup red or yellow bell pepper sliced

Serve as a dip with ½ cup sliced red or yellow bell pepper

7.13.2 PEPPERS & FRESH DILL SAUCE

Nutritional Information: *(½ cup veggie, 3 oz. protein)*

- ✓ ½ cup plain Greek yogurt
- ✓ ½ tsp. fresh dill chopped
- ✓ ¼ cup sliced cucumber
- ✓ ¼ cup red bell pepper sliced

Mix plain Greek yogurt with fresh dill. Dip cucumber and bell peppers in dip.

7.13.3 SWEET POTATO CHIPS

Nutritional Information: *(½ cup = ½ cup carbs, ½ tbsp. fat)*

- ✓ 2 sweet potatoes or yams (thinly sliced)
- ✓ cinnamon or sea salt
- ✓ 1/2 tbsp olive oil

Lay slices on a baking sheet and lightly cover with olive oil, sprinkle with either cinnamon or sea salt (depending on your taste). Bake at 350-degress for 50 minutes. They come out sweet, and salty and crunchy! Yum! Now we are talking!

7.13.4 SWEET POTATOE FRIES

Nutritional Information: ½ cup = *(½ cup carbs, 1/2 tsp. fat)* (yams are less desirable as they get mushy)

- ✓ 2 medium sweet potatoes
- ✓ 1 egg white (*using only egg white will make them crispier)
- ✓ 2 tsp. olive oil
- ✓ ½ – 1 tsp. ground cumin and paprika
- ✓ 1–2 crushed garlic cloves
- ✓ ¼ tsp. sea salt and ground pepper

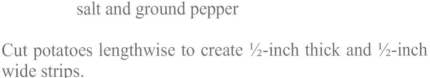

Cut potatoes lengthwise to create ½-inch thick and ½-inch wide strips.

NOTE: Keep the skin on for fiber and extra vitamins.

In a large bowl, whisk egg white until frothy. Whisk in oil, cumin, paprika, garlic, salt, and pepper. Add potatoes, tossing to coat. Spread on parchment-paper-lined, rimmed baking sheets.

Bake in top and bottom thirds of 425-degree oven for 30 to 35 minutes, (switch to bottom or top third of oven halfway through) until tender and edges are browned and crisp.

7.13.5 SPICY SALSA FRESCA

Nutritional Information: *(½ cup of this with veggies is ½ cup to 1 cup worth of veggies - way to go!)*

Pulse 1 jalapeno seeded
1 medium onion
Mix together in blender until minced

- ✓ Add 1½ pounds of Roma tomatoes (chopped)
- ✓ 2 cloves of garlic
- ✓ 4 tbsp. of fresh squeezed lime juice
- ✓ ½ cup fresh cilantro
- ✓ Salt and pepper to taste

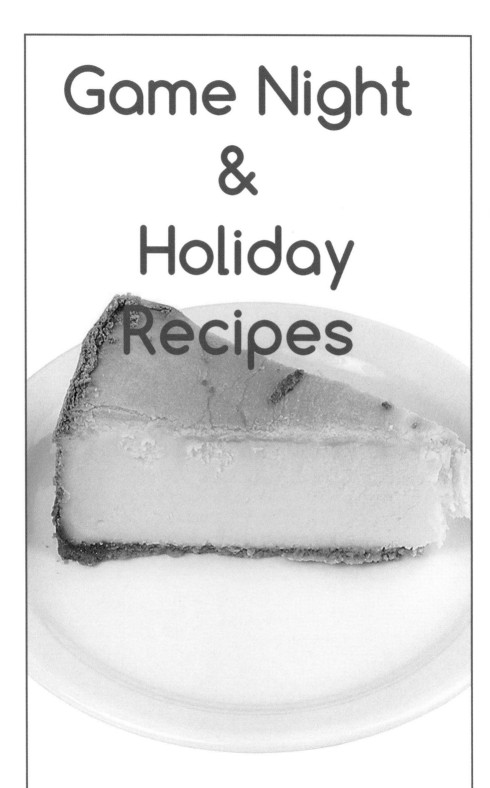

Game Night
&
Holiday
Recipes

7.14 Game Night & Holiday Recipes*
*these foods are to be eaten sparingly

7.14.1 BLACK BEAN NACHOS

Nutritional Information: *(3/4 cup = 1 cup carbs, 1 tbsp. fat, minimal veggies)*

- ✓ 2-6 ounce bags of baked pita chips
- ✓ 2 cups black beans rinsed and drained
- ✓ ½ cup light Monterey jack cheese or cheese of choice
- ✓ 4 tbsp. diced tomatoes
- ✓ 2 tbsp. red onion

Preheat oven to 350-degrees. Arrange chips in a single layer on two large ovenproof platters and top with equal amounts of beans, cheese, tomatoes, and onion. Bake for 5-10 minutes, and then garnish with cilantro and avocado if you desire.

7.14.2 PUMPKIN CHEESECAKE

Nutritional Information: 1 serving = *(3 oz protein, 1 tbsp. fat, trace carbs)*
Makes 6 servings

Crust:
- ✓ 1½ cup finely chopped walnuts
- ✓ 2 tbsp. coconut oil
- ✓ 2 tbsp. honey

Press all the above ingredients together and press in the bottom of your pie pan.

NOTE: It will seem not fully compact, but once you add pie filling, it all comes out nicely after cooked.

Filling:
- ✓ 8 oz. low fat cream cheese
- ✓ 8 oz. plain Greek yogurt
- ✓ ½ cup 100% pure maple syrup
- ✓ 1/3 cup pureed pumpkin
- ✓ ½ tsp. vanilla
- ✓ ¼ tsp. cinnamon and nutmeg

Blend until smooth, pour into piecrust and bake for 50 minutes at 350-degrees.

7.14.3 CREAMY CLEAN CHEESCAKE

Nutritional Informational: *(1 slice = 43 oz. protein, 1 tbsp. fat)*

Makes 4 slices

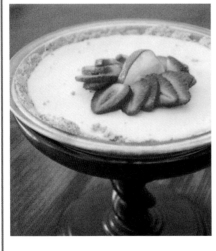

- ✓ 8 oz. cottage cheese
- ✓ 8 oz. plain Greek yogurt
- ✓ ½ cup 100% maple syrup
- ✓ 1 tsp. vanilla

Blend until smooth, pour in to piecrust under pumpkin cheesecake recipe, and bake for 50 minutes at 350-degrees. You can top this with your favorite fresh fruit topping or eat plain.

7.14.4 BAKED LIME WINGS

Nutritional Information: *(3 wings = 3 oz. protein, ¼ cup veggies)*

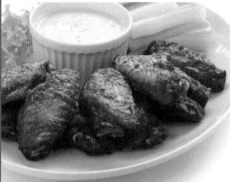

- ✓ 24 chicken wings
- ✓ 6 tomatillos diced (mix in blender)
- ✓ 1 tbsp. fresh lime juice
- ✓ ¼ cup low sodium soy sauce
- ✓ 3 tbsp. chopped cilantro

Bake wings in 375-degrees for approximately 25 minutes. Toss cooked chicken in sauce until coated, serve immediately. Use for party or for lunch/dinner, serves 12.

LUNCH & DINNER RECIPES

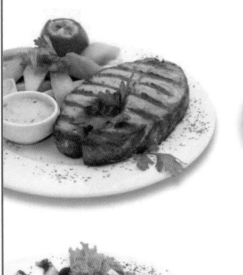
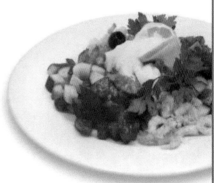
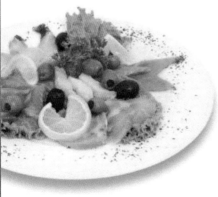
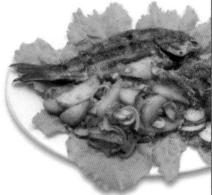

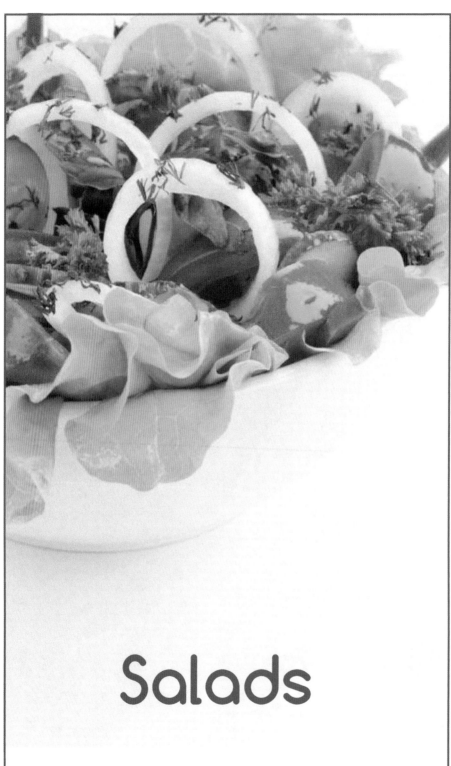

Salads

LUNCH & DINNER

When preparing lunch and dinner recipes be aware of the "free foods" on the exchange list. Get creative with spices and herbs to add variety and flavor. When dining out, a simple rule of thumb is to order a meat choice from the shopping list, add a side of cooked yam, brown rice and then your choice of veggies. Most restaurants will have these ingredients so you can stay on track.

Nutritional Information: *(3 oz. lean-protein, 1/2 cup carbs, 1/2 cup veggies)*

FREE FOODS: Balsamic vinegar, mustard, mushrooms, herbs, spices, among others. See Chapter 6 for shopping and exchange list.

7.15 Salads

Salads can be so delicious! There are so many ways to spice up a salad to make a flavor explosion. Spice up any salad with these main ingredients. Choose 5 of them:

- ✓ ½ cup dark green lettuce, spinach, kale, etc.
- ✓ Top with 3 oz. lean chicken, turkey, salmon, or 2 oz. meat
- ✓ 1 oz. cottage cheese (I love cottage cheese in place of dressing, so good!)
- ✓ Good flavorful fats: Top with 1/8 cup almonds, ½ avocado, or ¼ cup hummus
- ✓ 1 tbsp. olive oil with lemon juice or balsamic vinegar

Add various veggies:

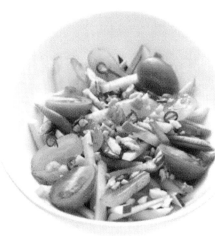

- Carrots
- Tomatoes
- Peppers
- Mushrooms

Add various fruits:

- Watermelon
- Grapes
- Apples
- Cranberries

Do not forget to add herbs!

- Basil
- Cilantro

Basil and Cilantro are my favorites and add major kick to any salad.

7.15.1 GRAPEFRUIT, AVOCADO, SALMON SALAD

Nutritional Information: *1 salad=(1 tbs. fat, 3 oz. protein, ¼ cup fruit, ½ cup veggie)*

Makes 4 salads

- ✓ 3 salmon fillets
- ✓ 1 Grapefruit
- ✓ 2 cups Arugula
- ✓ 1 Avocado
- ✓ Fresh lemon juice

Wrap salmon fillets individually in aluminum foil and bake for 30-35 minutes. Peel and segment grapefruit, reserve any juice in a bowl. Toss grapefruit with 2 cups of arugula and 1 sliced avocado with remaining juice. Top with 4 oz. wild salmon fillets. Divide all fish equally and salad mix.

7.15.2 ASPARAGUS SALAD

Nutritional Information: *(½ cup veggies, 2 oz. protein)*

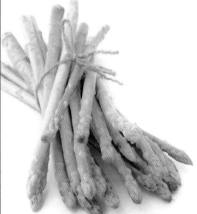

- ✓ 4 asparagus spears (cut into 2-inch pieces)
- ✓ 1/2 cup dark greens
- ✓ 1 hard-boiled egg
- ✓ 1 garlic clove minced
  - ✓ 1 tbsp. vinegar, salt and pepper to taste

Sauté asparagus with 2 tsp. olive oil or non-stick spray and one minced garlic clove. Boil egg for approx. 10 min. Place on top of ½ cup of dark greens, add chopped hardboiled egg, 1 tbsp. vinegar, salt and pepper to taste.

7.15.3 PEANUT BUTTER SALAD

Nutritional Information: *(½ cup veggies, ½ tbsp. fat)*

- ✓ ½ tbsp. natural peanut or almond butter
- ✓ 1½ tbsp. warm water (whisk together until smooth)
- ✓ ½ cup mixed greens

✓ 2 tbsp. raisins

Whisk peanut butter and water together. Toss with mixed greens and raisins.

NOTE: You can always add chicken or any meat source that sounds good for your protein. Also, chia seeds and raw nuts can be added as protein sources.

17.5.4 GRAPEFRUIT SUMMER SALAD

Nutritional Information: *(½ cup veggies, 1/2 tbsp. fat, ½ cup fruit)*

✓ ½ cup lettuce of any kind
✓ ½ avocado, sliced
✓ ¼ cup grapefruit cut into section
✓ ¼ cup fresh strawberries
✓ 1 tsp. sweet vinegar and grape seed oil

Line your salad plate with lettuce. Lay avocado, grapefruit, and strawberries over salad and sprinkle lightly with dressing.

NOTE: This great salad is perfect on those hot summer days when everything sounds heavy and cooking sounds hot. Try this out and stay on track with your goals.

NOTE: You can always add chicken or any meat source that sounds good for your protein. Also, chia seeds and raw nuts can be added as protein sources.

7.15.5 DELICIOUS APPLE SALAD

Nutritional Information: *(½ cup veggies, 1 tbsp. fat, ½ cup fruit)*

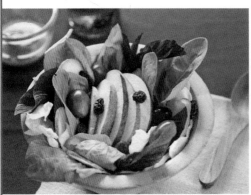

- ✓ ½ cup dark mixed greens of your choice
- ✓ 1 tbsp. chopped cashews (or raw unsalted nut of your choice)
- ✓ ½ sliced green apple
- ✓ 1 tbsp. apple cider vinegar

Combine ingredients.
NOTE: You can always add turkey or chicken for protein. Also, chia seeds and raw nuts can be added as protein sources.

7.15.6 FIESTA SALAD

Nutritional Information: *(3 oz protein, ½ cup veggies, 1/4 cup carbs, 1 tbsp. fat)*

- ✓ ½ cup romaine lettuce (you could use any salad greens you prefer)
- ✓ 3 oz. cooked chicken breast
- ✓ ¼ cup canned black beans (rinsed and drained)
- ✓ ½ chopped avocado
- ✓ 1/8 cup chopped tomatoes
- ✓ ½ fresh lime (squeezed)

Mix all together and enjoy!

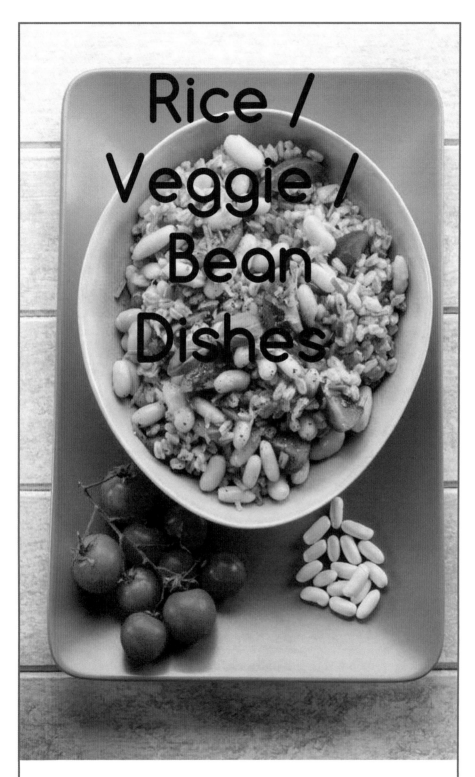

Rice /
Veggie /
Bean
Dishes

7.16 Rice / Veggie / Bean Dishes

7.16.1 VEGGIE SIDE DISH

Nutritional Information: *(½ dish = ½ cup to 1 cup veggies)*

- ✓ 2 spears of asparagus
- ✓ ½ cup broccoli
- ✓ 1 minced garlic clove
- ✓ 1 tsp. olive oil
- ✓ 2 tsp. lemon juice

Sprinkle asparagus and broccoli with 1 tsp. of olive oil and minced garlic, salt and pepper, and roast them in the oven at 400 deg. until they get a little crispy. Take them out and drizzle with 2 tsp. of lemon juice.

7.16.2 WARM SPINACH & QUINOA SALAD

Nutritional Information: *(½ cup = ½ cup veggies, ½ cup carbs, 1 tbsp. fat)*

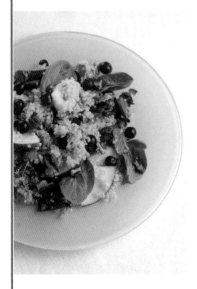

- ✓ 1½ cup quinoa
- ✓ 1 lb. baby spinach
- ✓ 1/2 c red wine vinegar
- ✓ 1/3 cup olive oil
- ✓ 4 oz. crumbled feta (optional)
- ✓ Salt & pepper to taste (coarse) (optional)

Cook quinoa with 3 cup water, bring to boil, cover, & simmer for 15-20 minutes. Whisk together red wine vinegar, olive oil.

Top warm quinoa with spinach and liquid mixture. Top with feta and salt and pepper (optional).

NOTE: Quinoa is a great carb because of its protein capabilities and as a main dish.

7.16.3 CURRY QUINOA

Nutritional Information: 1/2 cup *(½ cup carbs, ½ cup veggies)*

- ✓ ¼ cup quinoa
- ✓ 1/2 cup shredded carrots
- ✓ 2 tbsp. dried cranberries
- ✓ 1/4 cup canned chickpeas
- ✓ ½ tsp. curry powder

Cook quinoa according to package directions. Remove from heat, and let stand 10 minutes. Fluff with a fork and add ½ cup shredded carrots, 2 tbsp. dried cranberries, ¼ cup canned chickpeas and curry powder. Eat ½ cup as your starch option.

7.16.4 COWBOY CAVIAR

Nutritional Information: *(½ cup = ½ cup veggies, ¼ cup carbs, 1 tbsp. fat)*

- ✓ 2-15 oz. cans black beans (rinsed)

- ✓ 1-17 oz. can whole kernel corn (drained)
- ✓ 2 large tomatoes (chopped)
- ✓ 1 large avocado (diced)
- ✓ ½ red onion (chopped)
- ✓ ¼ cup chopped fresh cilantro

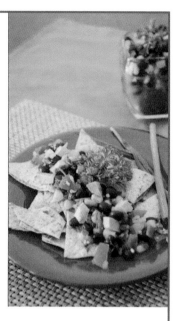

Dressing:

- ✓ 1 tbsp. red wine vinegar
- ✓ 1 clove garlic
- ✓ 1/8 tsp. cumin
- ✓ 3-4 tbsp. lime juice
- ✓ 2 tbsp. olive oil
- ✓ 1 tsp. salt
- ✓ ½ tsp. pepper

Combine all ingredients in bowl, cover and chill, and garnish with avocado slices or cilantro sprigs.

7.16.5 CHICKEN BASIL STIR FRY

Nutritional Information: *(3 oz. protein, 1/2 cup veggies)*

- ✓ 4 oz chicken
- ✓ 1 small serrano pepper
- ✓ 2 tbs. pad thai sauce
- ✓ 1/4cup cubed zucchini
- ✓ 1/4 cup red bell pepper

Spray pan or add 1 tsp. olive oil, zucchini, red bell pepper, 4 oz. chicken, and 1 small minced Serrano pepper, cook until chicken browns and pepper and zucchini are soft. Then add 2 tbs. pad thai sauce.

NOTE: Stir in ¼ cup fresh basil for extra flavor. Enjoy!

7.16.6 BEAN & VEGGIE SALAD

Nutritional Information: *(¾ cup = ½ cup carbs, ½ cup veggies, ½ tbsp. fat)*

- ✓ 2 -15 oz. cans chickpeas
- ✓ 3 red bell peppers (diced)
- ✓ 1 cup cilantro (chopped)
- ✓ 1 cup flat leaf parsley (chopped)
- ✓ 3 cloves garlic
- ✓ 1 Tbsp. olive oil

Combine all ingredients, and add lemon and sea salt to taste.

> Salads can be fun! Get creative by adding chia seeds, quinoa, a variety of nuts, berries, apples and pears.

7.16.7 3 BEAN SALAD

Nutritional Information: *(½ cup = ½ carbs/protein, 1 tbsp. fat)*

- ✓ 1-15 oz. can cannellini beans, rinsed and drained
- ✓ 1-15 oz. can kidney beans, rinsed and drained
- ✓ 1-15 oz. can garbanzo beans, rinsed and drained

- ✓ 1 cup fresh, finely chopped flat-leaf parsley
- ✓ 1 tbsp. fresh, finely chopped rosemary
- ✓ ½ red onion, chopped

Dressing:

- ✓ 1/3 cup apple cider vinegar
- ✓ 1 tbsp. honey
- ✓ ¼ cup olive oil
- ✓ 1 ½ tsp. salt
- ✓ ¼ tsp. black pepper

Mix the above ingredients together. Mix the dressing together and pour and mix together with first ingredients. Done in 10 minutes!

NOTE: Great dish to make and have in your fridge for a grab and go meal or snack!

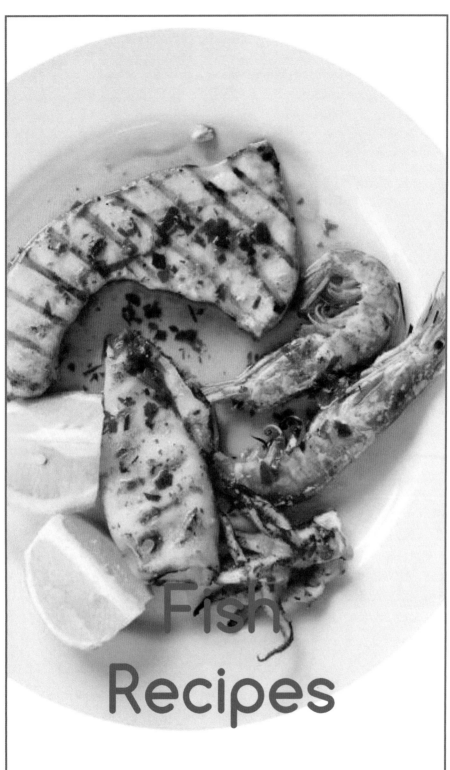

Fish
Recipes

7.17 Fish Recipes

7.17.1 SOUTHWESTERN GRILLED TUNA

Nutritional Information: *(3 oz. protein, ¼ cup fruit, ¼ cup veggies)*

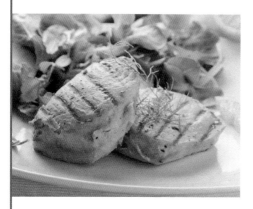

- ✓ 4 oz yellow fin tuna fillet
- ✓ 1/4 tsp. chili powder
- ✓ 1/4 tsp. ground cumin
- ✓ 1/4 tsp. pepper
- ✓ 1 tsp. olive oil sprinkle with

Brush yellow tuna with olive oil, chili powder, ground cumin and pepper. Grill until desired doneness. Top with ¼ cup fresh salsa recipe and serve with a cantaloupe wedge.

7.17.2 TILAPIA WITH RICE PILAF & SUGAR SNAP PEAS

Nutritional Information: *(3 oz. protein, ½ cup carbs, ½ cup veggies)*

- ✓ 3 oz tilapia fillet
- ✓ pkg. rice pilaf
- ✓ 1/2 cup sugar snap peas

Cook tilapia in 1 tsp. olive oil (dash of sea salt and black pepper) for approx.3 min. on each side. Tilapia will flake easily with a fork when done. Then prepare rice pilaf as directed on package. Place 1/2 cup rice pilaf and 1/2 cup steamed sugar snap peas on side of tilapia. Serve up a sophisticated meal in minutes.

Sandwiches and Wraps

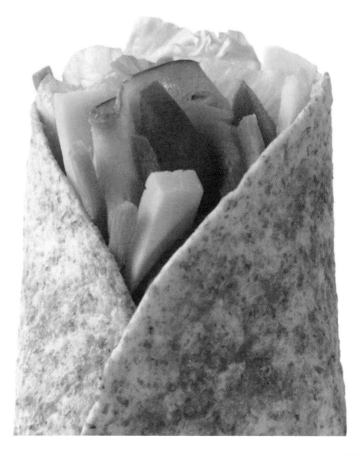

7.18 Sandwiches and Wraps

7.18.1 SANDWICH ROUNDS

NOTE: These are great as buns for your hamburger, or used as a sandwich. I like eating them on cold mornings with my healthy hot chocolate recipe.

Nutritional Information: *(1 2-3 inch round = 2 oz. protein, 1 tbsp. fat, ½ cup carbs)*

Makes about 6 pancake sized bread rounds

- ✓ 2 ½ cups (240g) almond flour
- ✓ 1 tsp. baking soda
- ✓ 1 cup (57g) yogurt (or coconut milk or almond milk)
- ✓ ¼ cup (60ml) unsalted butter or coconut oil
- ✓ 3 large eggs
- ✓ 2 tbsp. honey or maple syrup

Grease or spray a cookie sheet. Spread mixture in a round 2-3 inch diameter or size that you want. Spread mixture fairly thin, like you would be making crepes or thin pancakes. Bake at 350 for 15 minutes.

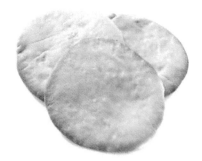

7.18.2 TURKEY PITAS

Nutritional Information: 1 serving= *(3 oz. protein, ½ cup veggies, ½ cup carbs)*

Serves 4

- ✓ 4 iceberg lettuce wedges
- ✓ 1 Ib. extra lean turkey burger
- ✓ 1 chopped bell pepper
- ✓ ½ onion diced
- ✓ 1 cup salsa (store bought or homemade recipe)

Sauce:

- ✓ 1 tbsp. apple cider vinegar
- ✓ 1 tbsp. extra virgin olive oil
- ✓ 1 tsp. cumin
- ✓ 1 tsp. chili powder

Cook turkey burger, bell pepper, onion in skillet until burger is fully cooked. Approx. 10 minutes. While turkey burger is cooking, mix together the sauce ingredients. Once turkey is fully cooked, mix in the sauce and place in 1/2 whole wheat pita with 1/4 cup salsa.

NOTE: You can have a side of ½ cup legumes or beans as your carb source or place them in the wrap.

7.18.3 FLAVOR POPPING SOUTHWEST WRAP

Nutritional Information: *1 wrap (½ cup carbs, ½ cup veggies)*

- ✓ 1 gluten free tortilla or lettuce wedge
- ✓ ½ cup shredded lettuce
- ✓ 1/3 cup black beans
- ✓ 2 tbsp. diced red onion & cilantro
- ✓ 1 tbsp. salsa
- ✓ Lime to taste

Place all ingredients in the gluten free tortilla or lettuce wedge and enjoy!

7.18.4 THAI LETTUCE WRAPS

Nutritional Information: 1 wrap = *(1 Tbsp. fat, 3 oz. protein, ½ cup of veggies)*

Makes 4 servings

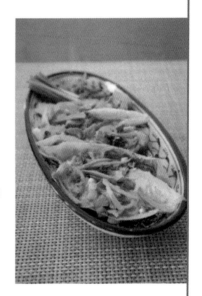

- ✓ 12 oz cooked chicken
- ✓ 2/3 cup creamy peanut butter
- ✓ ½ cup lite coconut milk or almond milk
- ✓ 1/3 cup orange juice
- ✓ 1-2 tbsp. red curry paste or curry powder
- ✓ 1 tsp. fresh minced ginger
- ✓ ½ tsp. garlic (optional)
- ✓ 1 lime (juiced)

Cook chicken or buy prepared chicken breast (without additives). Mix chicken with all ingredients, then place into lettuce wrap and top with 1/3-1/2 cup veggies of your choice.

Suggestion of veggies: shredded or chopped bell peppers, carrots, green onions, oranges, peanuts, and cilantro.

NOTE: This is another one of my children's favorite, and I am amazed at how many veggies they are consuming when eating this dish. Once again, the proof that peanut butter makes most things taste better.

7.18.5 SAVORY HUMMUS AND VEGGIE WRAP

Nutritional Information: *(½ cup carbs, 1 tbsp. fat, 2 oz. protein due to the hummus, ½ cup veggies)*

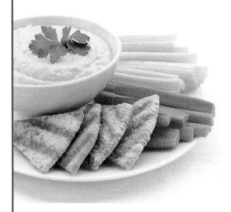

- ✓ 1/2 gluten free pita or lettuce wrap
- ✓ ¼ cup hummus
- ✓ 1/3 cup baby salad greens
- ✓ 4 slices of cucumber
- ✓ 1 bell pepper sliced

Mix and enjoy!

NOTE: I love pine-nut hummus.

7.18.6 MEXICAN BOWL

Nutritional Information: 1 = *(2 oz. protein, ½ cup veggies, ½ cup carbs, 1 tbsp. fat)*

Makes 4 servings

- ✓ 8 oz. chopped chicken breast
- ✓ 2 red bell peppers (cut into thin strips)
- ✓ 2 medium zucchinis (cut into thin strips)
- ✓ 1 ½ cup pinto or black beans
- ✓ 1 avocado and fresh salsa (optional)(sliced)

Coat a nonstick pan with cooking spray. Over medium-high heat, sauté the peppers and zucchini for about 7 minutes, then divide the pinto/black beans into four portions and place all ingredients in separate bowls.

Top with a quarter of the veggie mixture, a quarter of the avocado, and three tablespoons of salsa. Top with fresh cilantro and lime juice (optional).

7.18.7 TUNA PITA SANDWICH

Nutritional Information: ½ a sandwich = *(½ cup carbs, 3 oz. protein)*

- ✓ ½ gluten free pita or iceberg lettuce wedge
- ✓ 3 oz. tuna in water
- ✓ 2½ tbsp. plain Greek yogurt
- ✓ 1 tsp. Dijon mustard or regular
- ✓ 1 tsp. fresh chives
- ✓ ¼ cup diced fennel

Mix ingredients and place inside a gluten free pita or iceberg lettuce wedge.

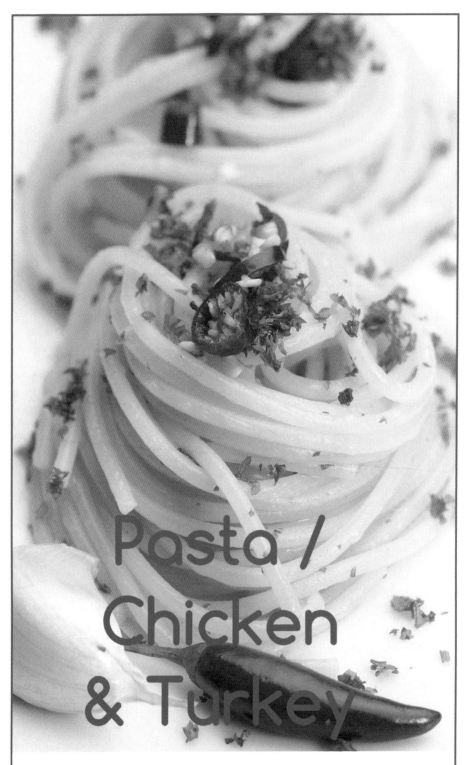

Pasta /
Chicken
& Turkey

7.19 Pasta / Chicken & Turkey Bake Recipes

7.19.1 SUMMER SQUASH & CHICKEN

Nutritional Information: *(½ cup veggies, 3 oz. protein)*

- ✓ 3 oz. cooked chicken
- ✓ 1/2 cup sliced squash and zucchini

Sauté, ½ cup sliced squash and zucchini, and 3 oz. chicken chunks until fully cooked. Approximately 10 min. Top with desired spices (my go to spice is curry or fresh rosemary with mustard).

NOTE: I love marmalades (awesome, tasty, fresh, and easy). I top with 1 Tbsp. of fresh herb marmalades.

7.19.2 EASY TURKEY DINNER

Nutritional Information: *(3 oz. protein ½ cup veggies)*

- ✓ 3 oz. ground lean turkey burger
- ✓ ½ onion
- ✓ 1 red pepper diced or sliced

In a skillet place turkey burger, onion and red pepper. Saute and add as many spices or herbs you would like from the shopping list. Cook until turkey is brown and thoroughly cooked. Approximately 10 minutes.

7.19.3 CHICKEN & MUSHROOM BAKE

Nutritional Information: *(3 oz. protein)*

- ✓ 3 oz. chicken breast

✓ 2 large Portabella mushrooms (sliced)

Coat a baking pan with non-stick spray or line with aluminum foil. Sprinkle non-salt spices, garlic, Mrs. Dash, etc., all over chicken and mushrooms, (mushrooms are a free food, so is mustard). Bake 30 minutes at 350-degrees.

NOTE: I made this dish every week leading up to the bikini world championships.

7.19.4 WARM EGG WHITE/SPINACH QUICHE

Nutritional Information: *(½ cup = 3 oz. protein, ½ cup veggies, ½ Tbsp. fat)*

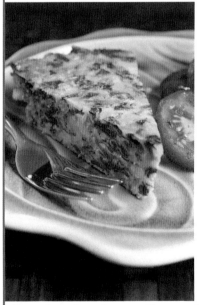

✓ ½ red onion chopped
✓ 8 oz. spinach around 2 ½ cup fresh
✓ 6 egg whites
✓ 2 gloves of garlic chopped fine (sauté in skillet)
✓ 1/4 cup feta cheese or 1/2 cup ricotta (optional)

Sauté spinach, garlic, and onion in skillet until spinach is wilted. Whisk together eggs and mix all together with cheese mixture. Add salt and pepper to taste and bake at 350-degrees for 30 minutes.

NOTE: You can also use whole eggs if you want.

7.19.5 CROCK POT DELIGHT

Nutritional Information: 1 cup =
(3 oz. protein, ½ cup carbs, ¼ cup veggies)

> If you know you are going to have a busy day. Take a few minutes to throw ingredients in your crock pot in the morning, turn it on and come home to a healthy, delicious dinner. Most weight loss plans are derailed due to lack of planning. It feels great to know that a healthy dinner is waiting for you after a long, busy day!"

- ✓ 1 lb. chicken
- ✓ 2 cans black beans
- ✓ 1 can diced tomatoes
- ✓ 1 cup brown rice
- ✓ 1 package taco season
  1 cup water

Place in crock-pot and cook for 6 hours.

7.19.6 DELICIOUS PASTA DISH

Nutritional Information: *(½ cup carbs, ½ cup veggies, 3 oz. protein, ½ tbsp. fat)*

- ✓ ½ cup gluten free pasta cooked or ½ cup cooked quinoa
- ✓ 3 oz. cooked chicken
- ✓ 2 tbsp. lemon juice
- ✓ 1/2 tbsp. olive oil
- ✓ ½ cup chopped basil
- ✓ ½ cup mushrooms

Sauté mushrooms, olive oil, and chicken together until mushrooms are lightly brown. Approx. 3-5 minutes. Place on top of cooked pasta and top with fresh basil and lemon juice.

7.19.7 CHICKEN PASTA

Nutritional Information: *(3 oz. protein, ½ cup veggies, ½ cup carbs)*

- ✓ 3 oz. grilled chicken
- ✓ 1/2 cup cooked gluten free pasta or ½ cup cooked quinoa
- ✓ ½ cup sautéed broccoli
- ✓ ½ tsp. orange zest
- ✓ 2 tbsp. extra virgin olive oil
- ✓ 1 minced garlic clove
- ✓ ½ tsp. red chili spice

Saute broccoli, chicken, olive oil chili spice, garlic, and orange zest together until chicken is fully cooked. Serve over pasta.

7.19.8 LEMON CHICKEN WITH GAZPACHO

Nutritional Information: *(3 oz protein, ½ cup veggies)*

Ingredients Chicken:

- ✓ 3 oz chicken breast
- ✓ 1 tbsp. olive oil
- ✓ ½ lemon squeezed
- ✓ 1 tsp. fresh rosemary

Ingredients Gazpacho:

- ✓ 1 cup stewed tomatoes

✓ 3 cloves garlic minced
✓ ½ cup chopped onion
✓ ¼ cup green pepper

Coat chicken with olive oil. Cover with lemon slices and rosemary and bake at 30° for 25 minutes. Combine Gazpacho ingredients in blender then serve ½ cup with chicken.

7.19.9 GREEK YOGURT CHICKEN SALAD

Nutritional Information: *(3 oz protein, ½ cup veggies)*

✓ 3 tbsp. plain Greek yogurt
✓ ½ tsp. mustard
✓ 2 tbsp. chopped celery
✓ 2.5 oz. cooked chicken chopped
✓ 1 tbsp chopped parsley and chives

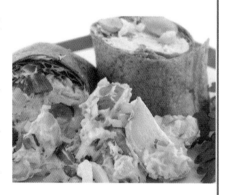

Mix all together and lay on ½ cup. chopped romaine lettuce.

7.19.10 SWEET AND SOUR CROCKPOT CHICKEN

Nutritional Information: *(1 cup = 3 oz. protein, ½ cup veggies)*

✓ 1 can low sodium natural chicken broth
✓ 1 can/jar sweet and sour mix (I like Trader Joes-less sugar and better ingredients)

- ✓ 2 chicken breasts cut up in bite sized chunks
- ✓ 1 cup broccoli, asparagus, or any other veggies you like (frozen or raw)

Cook in your crockpot for 4-6 hours on high. Quick, delicious easy meal to come home to for dinner.

Soup
Recipe

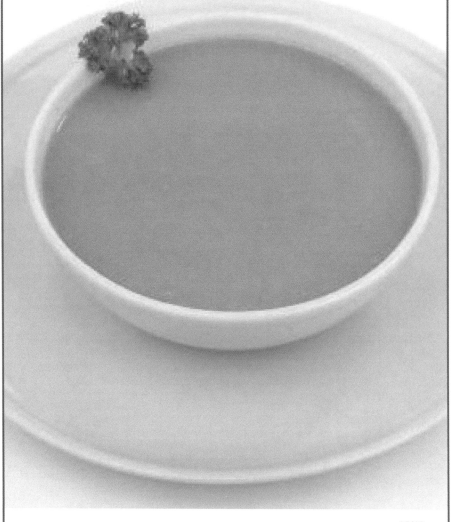

7.20 SOUP RECIPE

7.20.1 COCONUT PUMPKIN SOUP

Nutritional Information: *(1 cup with chicken = 3 oz. protein, ¼ cup carbs, ½ tbsp. fat)*

Makes 4 cups

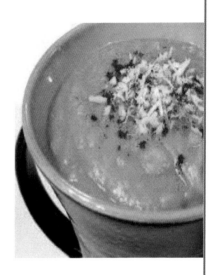

- ✓ 1 can chicken or veggie broth
- ✓ 1 14 oz. can lite coconut milk
- ✓ 1 15 oz. can pumpkin
- ✓ 2 cooked chicken breasts chopped
- ✓ 1 onion
- ✓ 1/2 tsp. cumin
- ✓ 2 tsp. curry
- ✓ 1/8 cup fresh ginger

Cook for 10 minutes. For your protein addition, you can add chopped cooked chicken to the end if you want. YUM!

7.20.2 BUTTERNUT SQUASH SOUP

Nutritional Information: *1 cup = ½ cup carbs, minimal veggies*

Ingredients for 1 oven cooked butternut squash:

- ✓ 2 tbsp. extra-virgin olive oil
- ✓ 1 onion, diced

- ✓ 1 tsp. shredded ginger root
- ✓ 4 cups oven cooked butternut squash
- ✓ 4 cups low-sodium chicken broth
- ✓ Salt/pepper to taste

To cook the squash, cut it length wise, take out the seeds and place in the oven on a cookie sheet, bake for aprox. 1 hour at 350 degrees (or you can buy frozen precooked squash). Heat oil in a large soup pot. Add onion and ginger and cook until softened. Add squash, onions, ginger, chicken broth and pulse/puree in blender. Add to large pot to reheat and salt and pepper to taste.

NOTE: To get your veggies, add a side of sautéed green beans or veggie of choice.

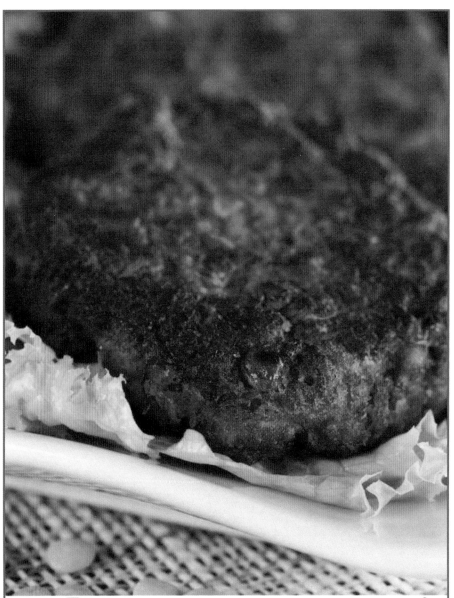

Burgers and Fish

7.21 Burgers & Fish

7.21.1 SANDWICH ROUNDS

NOTE: These are great as buns for your hamburger, or used as a sandwich. I like eating them on cold mornings with my healthy hot chocolate recipe.

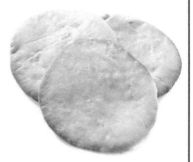

Nutritional Information: *(1 2-3 inch round = 2 oz. protein, 1 tbsp. fat, ½ cup carbs)*

Makes about 6 pancake sized bread rounds

- ✓ 2 ½ cups (240g) almond flour
- ✓ 1 tsp. baking soda
- ✓ 1 cup (57g) yogurt (or coconut milk or almond milk)
- ✓ ¼ cup (60ml) unsalted butter or coconut oil
- ✓ 3 large eggs
- ✓ 2 tbsp. honey or maple syrup

Grease or spray a cookie sheet. Spread mixture in a round 2-3 inch diameter or size that you want. Spread mixture fairly thin, like you would be making crepes or thin pancakes. Bake at 350 for 15 minutes.

7.21.2 TURKEY BURGER

Nutritional Information: *(3 oz. protein, ½ cup veggies)*

- ✓ 3 oz. extra lean turkey burger
- ✓ 1 tbsp. low sodium soy sauce
- ✓ ¼ cup sliced scallions
- ✓ 2 tsp. grated ginger

Form all ingredients into patty and grill 5 minutes on each side. Serve over a bed of ½ cup greens.

7.21.3 SALMON BURGER

Nutritional Information: *(1 burger = 3 oz. protein, ½ cup veggies)*
Makes 2 burgers

- ✓ 1 can wild Alaskan salmon
- ✓ 1 large egg white
- ✓ Spinach

Salt and pepper to taste, mix together the egg and salmon into patty, and then cook thoroughly on both sides, until fully cooked. Approximately 7 minutes on each side then lay burger on a bed of greens.

7.21.4 GREEK BURGER

Nutritional Information: 1 burger = *(3 oz. protein, ½ cup veggie) (leave out feta if you are not wanting the extra fat %)*

Take salmon burger recipe & top with

- ✓ ½ cup cucumber slices
- ✓ 1/8 cup feta cheese
- ✓ 1/2 cup greens

Place on top of a bed of greens.

7.21.5 FLAVORFUL TURKEY BURGER

Nutritional Information: 1 burger = *(3-4 oz. protein)*
Makes 4 burgers

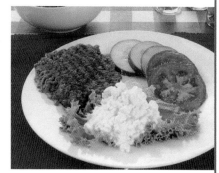

- ✓ 1 Ib. ground extra lean turkey burger
- ✓ 1 garlic clove minced
- ✓ ½ tsp. paprika
- ✓ ¼ tsp. ground cumin
- ✓ Salt and pepper to taste

Mix together, form into 4-inch patties, grill on medium-high until cooked through, approximately 7 minutes on each side.

7.21.6 BBQ BURGER

Nutritional Information: *(3- 4 oz. protein, ¼ cup veggies)*

- ✓ Use flavorful turkey burger recipe
- ✓ Top with sweet onion
- ✓ 1 Tbsp. low sugar BBQ sauce

Yum, yum…

7.21.7 GRILLED CHICKEN AND PINEAPPLE BURGER

Nutritional Information: *1 burger (3 oz. protein, ½ cup veggies, 1/8 cup fruit)*
Makes 2 burgers

- ✓ 2 boneless skinless chicken breasts
- ✓ 2 large pineapple slices
- ✓ ½ fresh jalapeno sliced
- ✓ ¼ red onion thinly sliced
- ✓ 2 slices Swiss cheese (*optional. Not recommended if needing to lose a lot of weight)

Grill chicken breasts, add cheese to breasts to melt right after cooked. Grill pineapple rings approx. 2 minutes per side. Top burger with pineapple, jalapeno and onions. Lay chicken on ½ cup of greens.

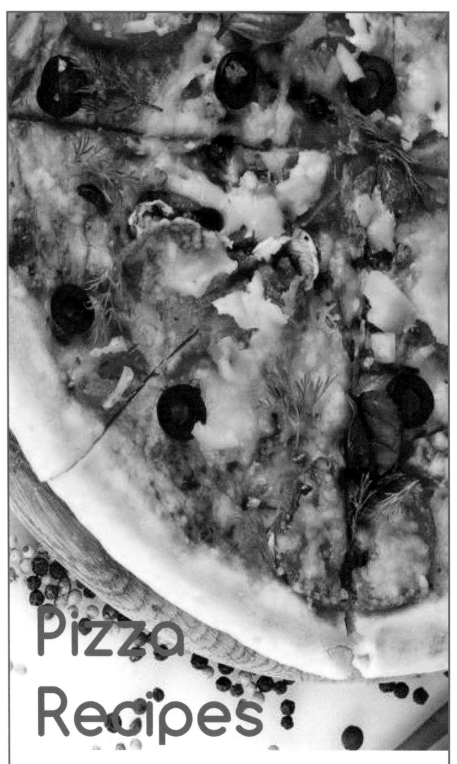

Pizza
Recipes

7.22 Pizza Recipes

7.22.1 PIZZA CRUST RECIPE

Crust:

- ✓ 1 cup buckwheat flour
- ✓ ¼ cup arrowroot powder
- ✓ ¼ teaspoon real salt
- ✓ 2 tbsp extra virgin olive oil
- ✓ 1 tbsp apple cider vinegar
  - ½ cup water

Mix together buckwheat flour, water and vinegar. If you've planned ahead, combine flour and vinegar and let sit for 12-24 hours. If not, preheat oven to 425 with pizza stone in oven for 30 minutes.

Stir in remaining ingredients until well mixed. The texture will be thinner than a standard crust. Place on pan in pizza crust form and bake on 400 degrees for 10 minutes. Take out and place toppings on, then bake your pizza for an additional 7-10 minutes at 350.

NOTE: When working with these ingredients, the dough may come out looking darker than regular crust.

7.22.2 COCONUT FLOUR PIZZA CRUST

- ✓ 1 cup shredded mozzarella cheese (*I use the full fat type)
- ✓ 1 egg
- ✓ 1 tbsp cream of buckwheat (or flax meal)
- ✓ 1 tbsp coconut flour

✓ 1/8 teaspoon baking soda

Preheat oven at 425. Mix all ingredients in a bowl until well combined. Line a cookie tray with parchment paper and spread the cheese mixture on the paper as thinly as possible, using the back of a spoon or fork.

Reduce heat to 400 and bake on the top rack for about 15 minutes or until the crust is starting to look golden in places. Remove from the oven and add desired toppings. Bake for a few minutes, just to melt cheese on top.

NOTE: This makes a crispier, delicious pizza crust.

7.22.3 BASIL & TOMATO PIZZA

Nutritional Information: *1 slice (½ cup carbs, ½ cup veggies, 2 oz. protein)*

Makes 3 servings

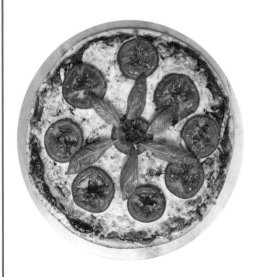

✓ 14 oz. pizza crust (*choose your pizza crust from above recipes or buy a gluten free one)
✓ ½ cup shredded part skim mozzarella cheese
✓ 1½ oz. prosciutto or lean ham

- ✓ ¾ cup sliced tomatoes
- ✓ 2 large garlic cloves minced
- ✓ ½ cup fresh basil
- ✓ Crushed pepper to taste

Cook at 350-degrees until crust is crispy.

NOTE: Cheese is optional. If you are looking to seriously lose weight eat it without the mozzarella Cheese.

7.22.4 CREATIVE PIZZA

Nutritional Information: *(3 oz. protein, ½ cup carbs, and ½ cup veggies)*

- ✓ 1 homemade pizza crust or gluten free/wheat free pita or tortilla
- ✓ ¼ cup tomato sauce
- ✓ ½ cup favorite veggies
- ✓ 3 oz. cooked lean spicy turkey burger (optional)

Sprinkle feta or low fat mozzarella on top.
Bake at 350-degrees for 7 minutes.

7.22.5 SOUTHWESTERN PIZZA

Nutritional Information: 1 serv. = *(½ carbs, ¼ cup veggies, 1 tbsp. fat)*

Makes 3 servings

- ✓ 12-inch pizza crust preference from recipes or buy a premade gluten free one
- ✓ 1 cup tomato salsa
- ✓ 1 1/3 cup canned black beans

- ✓ 1 small red pepper diced
- ✓ 2 scallions thinly sliced
- ✓ ¼ cup cilantro leaves

Place all ingredients on top of pizza crust. Bake at 450-degrees for 8-10 minutes.

7.22.6 PESTO PIZZA

Nutritional Information: *(1¼ cup carbs, 1½ cup veggies, 1 tbsp. fat)*

- ✓ 1 gluten free pita
- ✓ 2 tsp. pesto
- ✓ ½ cup arugula
- ✓ ¼ chopped tomato
- ✓ 1 tbsp. pine nuts
- ✓ 1 tsp. lemon juice

Place 2 tsp. on pita and broil in oven until golden. Approx. 2-5 minutes. Take out and top with remaining ingredients. Pepper to taste.

7.22.7 SAVORY VEGGIE PIZZA

Nutritional Information: 1 mushroom = *(½ cup veggies, 1 tbsp. fat)*

- ✓ Take 3 giant mushroom heads
- ✓ 1 onion or handful of shallots
- ✓ 3 cloves of garlic minced
- ✓ 3 tomatoes diced
- ✓ 1 chopped leek
- ✓ Squeeze juice of one lemon

✓ Dice 5 basil leaves

Cook onion, garlic, tomatoes, leek, and lemon together and place on top of mushrooms. Sprinkle with Romano cheese or leave plain, bake in a 400-degrees oven for 12 minutes.

Top with fresh basil leaves. The flavors pop in this delicious recipe.

7.22.8 MOUTHWATERING PROSCIUTTO & MUSHROOM PIZZA

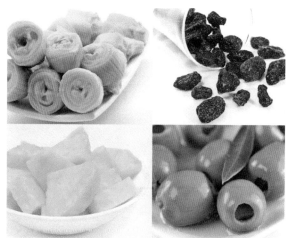

Nutritional Information: *(1 pita = 1 cup carbs, 2 oz. protein, ¼ cup veggies)*

✓ 1 gluten free pita
✓ low sodium chicken broth
✓ 6 shitake mushrooms
✓ 2 oz. prosciutto
✓ 1 tbsp. minced garlic
✓ ¼ tsp. red pepper flakes

Sauté mushrooms, prosciutto, garlic and pepper flakes, then cook with 1/3 cup low sodium chicken broth. Cook for 2-3 minutes (until liquid has almost evaporated).

Place mixture on top of pita and sprinkle with goat cheese and fresh basil. Broil 4 inches from heat for 1 minute, rotate, and broil 1 additional minute.

7.22.9 SARAH'S CHEESY PINEAPPLE PIZZA

Nutritional Information: *(½ cup carbs, ½ cup veggies, ¼ cup fruit)*

- ✓ Naan bread or gluten free pita bread
- ✓ 1/4 cup tomato sauce
- ✓ ¼ cup fresh pineapple
- ✓ 2 tsp. pizza or Italian seasoning
- ✓ 1/8 cup to ¼ cup low fat mozzarella cheese or feta (most kids do not like feta)

Take naan or gluten free pita, top with tomato sauce and seasoning, pineapple and cheese. Bake in the oven on 375-degrees for 8 minutes (until cheese melts and sauce is warm).

7.22.10 CHICKEN ARTICHOKE PIZZA

Nutritional Information: *(½ cup carbs, ½ cup veggies 3 oz. protein, 1 tbsp. fat)*

- ✓ Pre-made gluten free Naan bread or pita bread

- ✓ 1 tbsp. low fat Alfredo sauce
- ✓ 3 oz. cooked chicken
- ✓ ½ cup artichoke hearts
- ✓ 1/8 cup kalamata olives & feta cheese

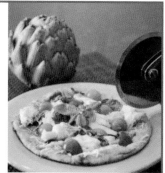

Top your naan bread or pita bread with alfredo sauce. Top with artichoke and chicken. Sprinkle feta cheese on top and bake it on 375-degrees for approximately 8 minutes (until cheese melts and sauce is warm).

Chapter Eight

Review of the Basic Rules

As we review the basic rules, I felt this was a good opportunity to discuss why each of us need to place "clean eating" in our lives as priority #1.

8.1 Why Clean Eating?

Clean eating is eating the way nature intended. You eat the foods our bodies evolved to function best on, and that makes you feel – and look – fantastic. When you eat clean, you eat more often. You will eat lean protein, complex carbs and healthy fats. These practices keep your blood-sugar levels stable and keep you satisfied.

Keep in mind the food list is not exhaustive; there are definitely other things that are healthy and beneficial, but for now, we will stay with the shopping list. Sometimes it takes a bit of fine-tuning. Work to have some patience and flexibility in the process. One thing for sure, no one benefits from eating sugar and this is the foundation and the basis for most processed foods.

See the benefits of eating clean below.

The benefits of eating clean are many:

- Elevated mood
- Increase circulation
- Decrease organ inflammation
- Repair scars, injuries, and wrinkles

- You will increase production of elastin and collagen
- Increased efficiency in metabolism, resulting in cellular repair

Learning HOW to eat (to be lean and fatigue free), and it will become second nature to you.

8.2 Review of the Basic Rules

- Eat every 2-4 hours (3 being ideal)
- Eat within an hour of awakening
- Include protein every time you eat to keep you full and energized
- Your veggies can be cooked (steamed, sautéed in cooking spray, roasted) or raw
- Do not WAIT until you are "hungry" to eat
- Water throughout the day keeps you healthy and hydrated (1 gallon per day is ideal)
- Be prepared and know when and where the next meal is coming from
- Log your food to know what is really happening
- Take one day at a time, making changes is a lifestyle change

Conclusions

I said this earlier, but…

I want everyone to have the tools to look and feel their best! I want to instill hope in everyone who has a desire to lose weight, have more energy and more self-love. I know that if I can bring confidence in one's mind and body, then it will translate into the world.

I know when someone feels good about himself or herself, each has more capacity to love, to get out and enjoy nature, to enjoy his or her families and friends. I know feeling good about one's self, creates better relationships with your spouse or partner, your family, friends, and associates.

As your openness grows, oneness with others increases, and your satisfaction in all your relationships increases ten-fold.

Metric Conversions

Yogurt Conversions

1 ounce = 28.34 grams, so one cup of yogurt weighs 227 grams.
1/4 cup of yogurt = 57 g
1/3 cup of yogurt = 76 g
1/2 cup of yogurt = 113 g

Dry Goods:

Flours

Cups	Grams	Ounces
1/8 Cup (2 tbsp)	16g	.563 oz
1/4 Cup	32g	1.13 oz
1/3 Cup	43g	1.5 oz
1/2 Cup	64g	2.25 oz
2/3 Cup	85g	3 oz
3/4 Cup	96g	3.38 oz
1 Cup	128g	4.5 oz

Rolled Oats

Cups	Grams	Ounces
1/4 Cup	21g	.75 oz
1/3 Cup	28g	1 oz
1/2 Cup	43g	1.5 oz
1 Cup	85g	3 oz

Helpful Math tips:

1 ounce = 28.34 grams
1 pound = .453 kilograms

1 g = .035 oz
1 kg = 2.2 lb
1 fluid oz = 29.57 milliliters

Baking Conversions for cups and tsp. and tbsp.

1 c. dark chocolate chips = 152 g
1 c. cocoa powder = 128 g
1 c. walnuts, chopped= 122 g
1 c. walnut/pecan halves= 99 g
1 c. shredded coconut= 71 g
1 c. coconut oil = 205 g
1tbsp. baking powder= 12 g
1 tbsp. salt = 18 g
1 tbsp. =14.79 ml
1 tsp. =4.92 ml

It is hard to convert weight to volume for example; measuring 1/2 c. veggies is going to be different in grams than 1/2 c. walnuts. I would recommend ordering some inexpensive measuring cups if that makes it easier for you.

Here are some math conversions to help you determine weight:

1 cup of Raw Broccoli weighs 91 grams.
91 divided by 28 grams equals 3.25 oz
So... 1 cup of Raw Broccoli weighs 3.5 oz
1 cup of Raw Spinach weighs 30 grams
30 divided by 28 grams equals 1.07 oz
So... 1 cup of Raw Spinach weighs 1.07 oz
1 cup of Chopped Tomatoes weighs 180 grams.
180 divided by 28 grams equals 6.42 oz
So... 1 cup of Chopped Tomatoes weighs 6.42 oz

This link can help you with some conversions:
www.onlineconversion.com

My love for fitness and health

- ✓ Top 10 World Bikini Championships
- ✓ Star in top fitness videos
  - Walmart
  - Sears
  - Target
- ✓ Worked alongside and on their products
  - GSP
  - Jillian Michaels
  - Kathy Smith
- ✓ Wrote the Nutrition book for *Rip 60*
- ✓ Wrote *Think and Be Slim*
- ✓ Executive to largest distributor World Fitness Equipment
- ✓ Studied pre-med and nutrition
- ✓ Trained over 1,000 individuals
- ✓ Fitness & Nutrition expert for NBC affiliate Studio 5
- ✓ Contributor to KUED TV *Speaking on Women's Health*
- ✓ Fitness model for US & Women's Health Magazine

What Danette Is Up To

Danette holds private retreats each year in beautiful Costa Rica. If you want to experience a total transformation for your body, heart, mind & soul in the natural, serene beauty of Costa Rica, click this link to learn more: www.mindfulhealthretreats.com

You can follow upcoming events and get free fitness & nutrition videos at:
www.danettemay.com

Be sure to connect with Danette on social media at the following links:

Facebook:
www.facebook.com/EatDrinkAndShrink
Pinterest: **http://pinterest.com/danettemay/**

We welcome your questions and comments. Please email us at **support@eatdrinkshrinkplan.com**

If you want to accelerate your goals and ensure you are maximizing your results when it comes to exercise, join Danette May in the Forever Fit Personal Training site. You will be shown exactly what to do to get lasting results with weekly workout videos that take only 20 min. or less, access to live telecals with Danette, additional fat burning recipes, and a community of likeminded friends. Go to **http://theforeverfitchallenge.com/monthly/.**